See citations in the back of this book for previous publication information.

Published in the US in 2025 by
CLEVO BOOKS
1026 Euclid Ave.
Cleveland, Ohio
44115
www.clevobooks.com

© 2025 James Dolbow, Michael Wynn, Douglas Hester, Brenda Butka, William Rogers, Brian Christman, Lealani Mae Acosta, and Veena Kumar.

All rights reserved. No part of this publication may be reproduced or transmitted in any form or by any means, electronic or mechanical, including photocopy, recording, or any information storage and retrieval system, without permission in writing from the publisher.

Library of Congress Control Number: 2024952038

ISBN: 978-1-68577-015-0

E-book ISBN: 978-1-68577-016-7

Printed in the USA
Cover art and design: James Dolbow
Interior layout: Ron Kretsch
First American Edition

Small Important Things
An Anthology of Modern Physician Poetry

Edited by James Dolbow D.O.

Featuring physician poets

Lealani Acosta M.D.
Brenda Butka M.D.
Brian Christman M.D.
James Dolbow D.O.
Douglas Hester M.D.
William Rogers D.O.
Veena Kumar M.D.
Michael Wynn D.O.

CONTENTS

JAMES DOLBOW

You Know I Love You, Right? 12
Last Call 13
Played Out 14
Pushing Water 15
Time 16
19 Beds 17
Please, Just Keep Her Comfortable 18
Curtain Call 21
Diagnosis of Exclusion 22
The Sound of Solemn 23
It's Time 24
In Sickness and in Health 25
To Save The World 26
Small Important Things 27
Mixed Feelings 28
Rinse. Repeat. 30
Unprepared 32
And There She Was 34
Sunset 36
Ode to the Intern 37
Pieces 38
Surprise 39
Tethered 40
The Way Willows Fall 41
A Child of Deaf Parents 42
The Luxury of Shame 43
Nostalgia 45
Call Me When You Get There 47
Complicit 48
For the Living 49
Folded 50
Apathy of Chronic Disease 51

Confession 52
The Space Between 53
Rhythmed One 55
Intractable 57
Standard of Care 58
What Matters Most 59
Room 1 60
Room 2 63
Entropy 65
Absent 66
These Talking Halls 67

MICHAEL WYNN

Advice to My Younger Self While Making Evening Rounds 70
Being Receptive 71
Evening Autopsy 72
It Starts with the Brain 73
Observations of a First Year Neurology Resident 74
Four Pieces of Advice for New Neurologists 75

DR. DOUGLAS HESTER

First Case with Adéle and Aegis 80
Spraying Cotton in Bolivar County, Mississippi, the Summer
Following My First Year of Medical School 81
Breaking-in 82
An Inquiry Concerning the Nature of the Clinical
Efficacy of Propofol on the Soul 83
Final Diagnosis 84
A Medical Practice 86

DR. BRENDA BUTKA

Do Not Resuscitate 90
Shift Change in Bedlam 92

Traveling Light 94
Dear Abby 96
Diagnosis: M. avium, hepatitis C, carcinoma,
thrombocytopenia, hemoptysis 99
Charting in Clinic 100

DR. WILLIAM ROGERS

Agonal..106
Elevator Poem #9 107
some biutiful swallow..108
Pick Up the Phone 113
Hospital Gift Shop..114
Can't You Just Care..116
It's Okay, You're Okay..117
Rescue Kit for Junkie 119
Ride Home with Me Later 120
Patient Lost to Follow Up***..122

DR. BRIAN CHRISTMAN

CCU Jazz 126
Resilience...127

DR. LEALANI MAE ACOSTA

Spaghetti with Rice 130

DR. VEENA KUMAR

The Scent of Collapse 134
It's Christmas Eve 135
Life 136
Residency...137
Mr. X 139

Dedicated to our patients

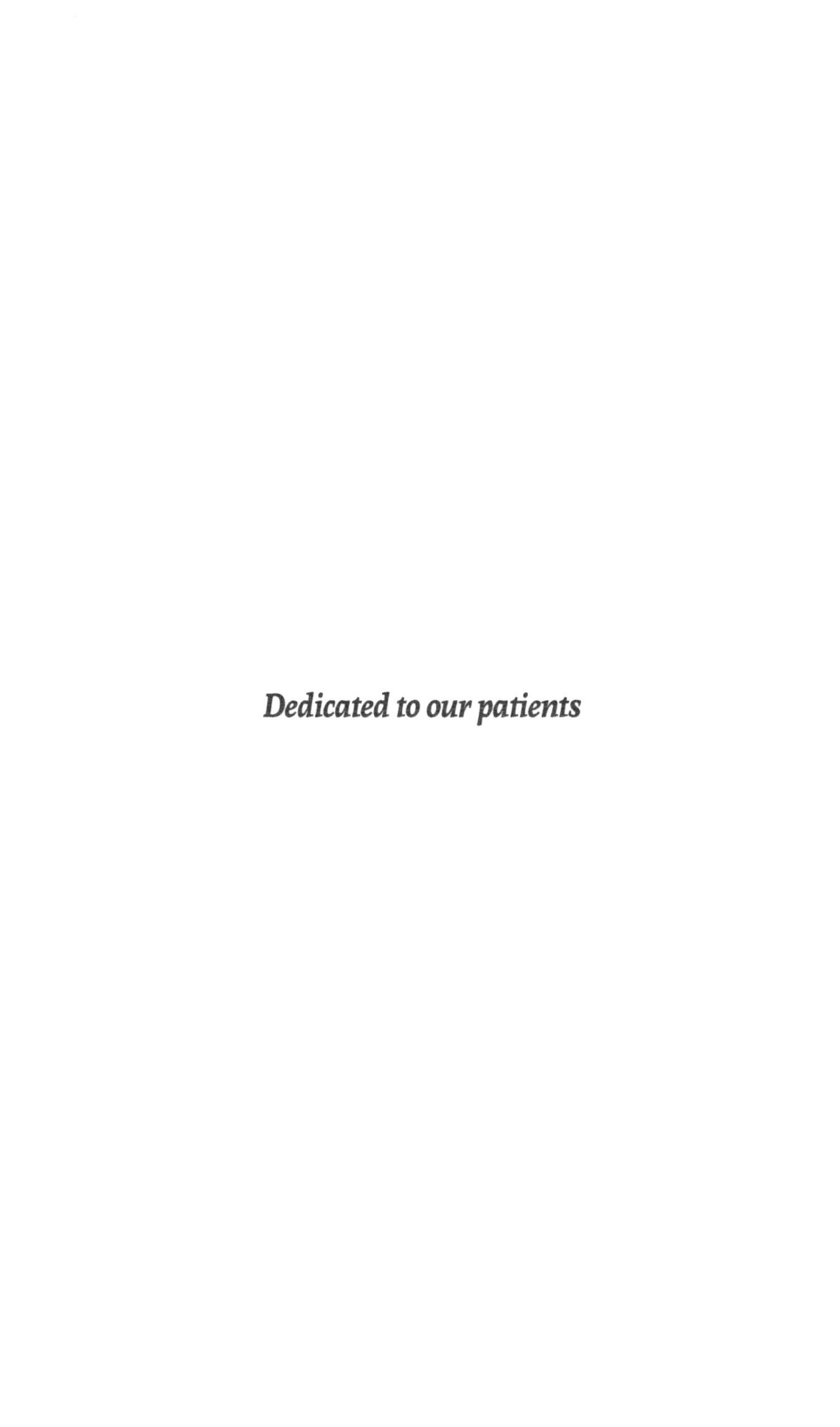

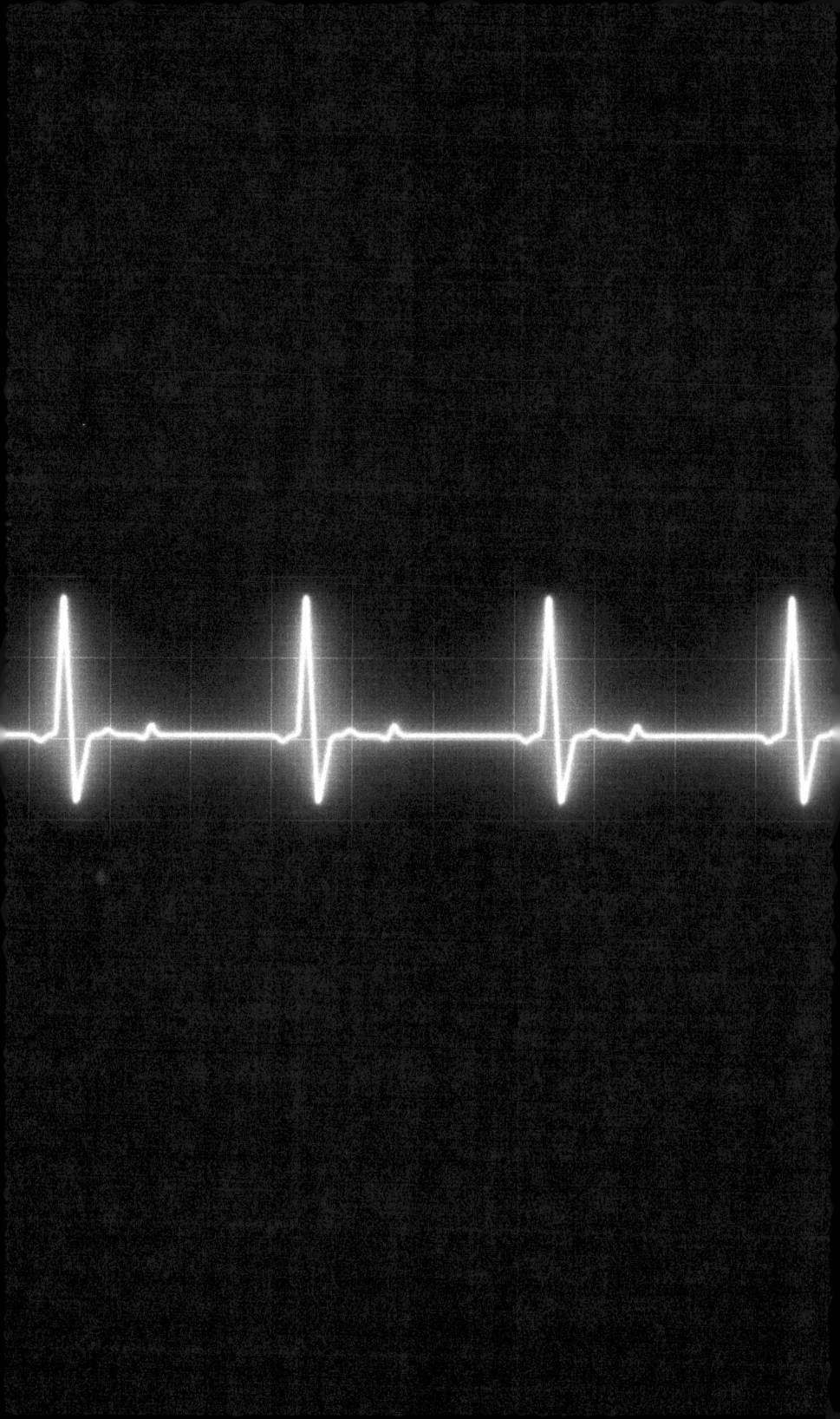

JAMES DOLBOW D.O.

Dr. James Dolbow is a board-certified neurologist and epileptologist at MetroHealth medical center in Cleveland, OH. Born in Nashville, TN, Dr. Dolbow graduated from Lincoln Memorial University College of Osteopathic Medicine in rural Harrogate, TN before moving to Cleveland for neurology residency and epilepsy fellowship.

Inspired by the deep interpersonal aspects of physicianhood, which are the focus of much of his writing, Dr. Dolbow's poetry explored the inner thoughts and feelings of the more serious, somber, and emotional situations common in hospitals and patient care. Working as a hospital janitor prior to attending medical school, his writing often comes from the perspective of others like patients, families, and non-physician care staff, with many of his pieces more resembling story-telling and introspection than formal traditional poetry. His first published poem, *You Know I Love You, Right?* explored the often overlooked lost close relationships of those with dementia. It was awarded the 2021 *American Academy of Neurology Award for Creative Expression of Human Values in Neurology*. Since that time Dr. Dolbow has been writing about the scenes and situations that inspire him during his training and in his medical practice, mainly the meaningful conversations with patients and families, the serious emotional situations of patient care, and life as a new physician. Dr. Dolbow is also the author of several other creative medically-related books including *The Neurology Riddle Book*, *The Neuroanatomy Riddle Book*, and *Intern Year: 20 Things You Didn't Learn in Medical School*. Most meaningful to him in this book is the ability to co-write several poems with his creative writing mentor and close personal friend Dr. William Rogers.

YOU KNOW I LOVE YOU, RIGHT?

76-year-old man: "Memory Problems"
An agreeable face warm with energy.
An endearing smile below a wrinkled forehead.
"My wife here wants my memory checked," he shrugs.
"She says I'm forgetting things. I think she's overreacting."
Their fingers intertwine where they fit best.
The pattern on their socks match.
Looks at her with an adoring stare.
Back to me with a hint of fear.
With his other hand, the fingers pale.
Pressing into the fabric at his knee.

79-year-old man: "Follow-up Memory Problems"
A slow glance up and then back down to the floor.
Wife with red eyes holds his left hand.
Tightly between her two.
"It's getting worse," she says.
"I don't think the medicine is working."
He looks at her.
Squeezes her hand.
"I'm so sorry, my love," he cries.

84-year-old man: "Weight Loss, Follow-up Memory Problems"
A distant gaze.
A kind and gentle, slow smile.
Red, sleep-deprived wife's eyes. The pattern of fractured glass.
Voice trembling, she asks, "Is he still in there?"
She begins to cry.
Quiet. His socks bunched about his ankles.
"I love you so much," she says desperately.
He gazes up at her. Eyes distant. Hands together. Gentle smile.
No response.
Adjusting to face him, tearfully she asks,
"You know I love you, right?"

LAST CALL

Smoky-eyed unshaven face,
punished with years lost
chasing that never-ending last drink,
and final pack
that brought him here
to his closing ceremony.

Dirt rimmed nails
ending fingers neat with yellow
cracked skin meeting chapped muddled palms.
A faded tattoo playing taps
to his brothers left on the battlefield.

Two ex-wives and three kids
with heads and hats hung on hope,
decayed after years of betrayal,
and long nights spent wishing to be
prioritized over a final pint.

Now watch him die
through daily updates from a
doctor who doesn't even know him,
each ripe with apathy,
let free with today's last call.

PLAYED OUT

But that's the dark matter of it.
The perfect emphasis on flawed diction,
played out over decades of
a daydreamed career.
Slowly become aggressively mediocre
with no windows.
A career that breathes desperately into
a leaking paper bag filled
with new combinations of
old hats, and a carrot dangling a stick.
Copy-forwarding
rounding coffee death notes,
while listening with empty ears
to the pills roll in the palms
of their own smeared ink.

PUSHING WATER

Standing,
watching,
moving water from one place
to another.
First bucket, then mop,
then floor.

He notices the patterns in patterns
around him.

His day starts here,
in this same spot,
everyday,
and ends here,
in this same spot,
everyday.
This same spot.

Head down,
painting the floor,
east to west,
everyday.
Following the sun.

While hospital workers kick through the
coffin nails and dead skin
that line the textured walls
and scarred tiles
stained with the dragged feet of transients,
and lifers

While scared patients beg
for sips of water
through lips crusted with stale sleep

And some kid
plays chopsticks
on the lobby piano.

TIME

To come home and see my
girl, twelve years older
than the last time
I looked up.

Bubble wrap and tic tac toe,
hidden candy.
Floor sits now couch sits
once a year.
Play time now gone,
and closeness fallen
far from the tree.

We used to hide under
kitchen tables,
and play with stickers,
and make necklaces,
and talk about your day.

And now I trade family
for strangers,
everyday.
Every minute.
Every excuse.
For what?

We used to pet the dog together,
and play dress up,
and make up,
and tea party.

You would walk around in
my big leather shoes
and we would play
doctor,
and you would listen to
my heart.

19 BEDS

19 beds
In 19 rooms,
arranged in ascending order,
in a square-shaped ward.

Halls filled with coats and scrubs.
Each with teeth
first lost, then regrown,
and now cut
working in a system much larger than themselves,
but equally broken.
A collective shoelace
untied and tripped on.

An unsorted pile
of medical record numbers,
families tired of praying.
Graham crackers and ginger ale.

But these 19 rooms are sacred.
Filled with memories of battles lost and won,
and peppered with a patinaed grace
only we can see.

PLEASE, JUST KEEP HER COMFORTABLE

Please doctor,
just keep her comfortable.
I've looked at her for so long now,
trying to find her.
Like a blizzard,
we're on opposite sides of.
Any sign of
the woman I love
missing in the white of the hospital.
The strongest woman I know.
My best friend.
The woman whose life and presence
sits at the center of my chest.

Good doctor,
just keep her comfortable.
I've kissed her every day for so long now.
I remember our first kiss.
My whole world changed
at the place where our lips met,
and touched forever.
To hold her was to swim
in the tide of her breathing lungs.
To share her heart's tempo.

Good doctor, please.
Christ, I miss her fingers
in mine warm, at home.
That perfect fit.
Her face makes a smile
when I close my eyes.
The woman who used to dance
and dance, a flame around the living room.
Embarrassing me.

I wish I stood up and danced with her more.
I wish I was more goofy with her,
when I had the chance.

Please doctor,
Just keep her comfortable.
Because I don't know
what my life is without her.
I miss her voice.
Sometimes when I walk
through the halls of our home,
I hear her.
Sometimes in this hospital room,
when it's completely silent
minus the hum of the heat vent,
the constant buzz of the artificial light
and the tireless beeps of machines,
wet drops of snow go down outside the window and
I hear her joke about getting old together,
and being senile enough
to hide our own Easter eggs.
We were supposed to lose marbles together,
and it makes me smile.
And I miss her so goddamn much.
And sometimes these memories make my tears
upturn to the contour of this goofy smile.
and I don't know
what my life will be without her.

Please Doctor,
as she lays here,
not spoken and barely moved in weeks,
can you please just keep her comfortable?
She means more to me
than you understand.
I need you to look at her and then look at me
and tell me

over and over again,
that you will keep her comfortable.
I need you to tell me she is not in pain.
I need you to tell me she is important to you.
I need you to tell me you understand.
I would die next to her if I could.
If you would let me.

So please doctor,
please keep her comfortable.
I need you to love her too.
I desperately need you to love her too.

CURTAIN CALL

She listens,
She listens,
but knows,
this is her life's closing.

And as her doctor
speaks softly,
with solemn words
brushed off
and reused
between dying patients,
she can hear the curtain pull,
and the crowd hush.
She can feel the lights dim.

She takes her bow.

A beautiful life closed.
Letting go her body,
so that it might be
brushed off
and reused.

This poem was co-written by Dr. James Dolbow and Dr. William Rogers.

DIAGNOSIS OF EXCLUSION

Shoes dirty, nails coarse
once blue shirt, now too faded
to see the logo.

Neglected, missing
teeth behind cracked, chapped lips
and curled untrimmed beard.

Shoulders high, strong, thin
from years of bags, shame, and sun
with head and eyes down.

How can I, a "have"
best show warmth, kindness, true love
to you, a "have-not?"

With a foam mattress,
mockingly colorful pills,
and a drawn curtain?

Or a cold sandwich,
weak, stale coffee, cream, sugar,
and one for the road.

THE SOUND OF SOLEMN

There's a sound for everything.
Many quiet, heard by few.

There is a sound of solemn.
Hushed but tactile.
Coming in many forms.
Heard beyond the rhymed beeps of hospital machines.
Beyond reports given and received.
A sound you feel in your lungs.

It's the sound of deep breaths,
eyes meeting the floor,
and long pauses.

It's the sound of a spouse's eyes
meeting yours,
and the description of a wake up stroke.

It's the sound of a guarded prognosis
and the sound of the grace of acceptance.

It's the sound of your love for your patient
and the quiet of the sorrow of her husband.

There is a sound for everything.
Many quiet, hushed, but tactile.

IT'S TIME

It's time.
Six people
half-circled around
a dying woman.
Some cry, crumble,
and withdraw.
Others stand, with arms crossed
or hands in pockets,
or on shoulders.

Air soft, grey with
whispered words of love
and mumbled regrets.

Some glare.
Bones ignited
at the sight
of the absence of my palms
pressing on their
mother's frail chest.

While others plan their outfit
for the funeral.

                                      Cry,
                                   crumble,
                                    stand,
                                  whisper.

                                  It's time.

IN SICKNESS AND IN HEALTH

Dear resident,

Remember where you're from.
> *The frayed grey snout of your stuffed elephant*

Remember your first patient.
> *that can't remember you,*

Remember why you're here.
> *dreaming loudly with fresh decoration,*

Remember who you were.
> *drunk on self-importance.*

Remember your successes.
> *The way your hand lived in hers,*

Remember your mistakes.
> *nightly walks, and the way she folded her laundry,*

Remember those that you watched die.
> *and in the calm of that cold room,*

Remember those you saved.
> *the last kiss you still live inside.*

Remember to eat.
> *What lived in the ribs of her ribs*

Remember to breathe.
> *was the last drop of air in the world,*

Remember to listen.
> *and a story told to itself in the dark,*

Remember to cry.
> *with nothing to have or to hold.*

Remember those you love.

TO SAVE THE WORLD

Purpose-filled shuffled feet,
shifting meds from one
mouth to the next.
Sleeves and hair up,
sorting the value of lives.
Rent paid in camaraderie.
Cold meals while standing.
Strangers treated like blood by day,
tiptoeing into homes
already asleep by night.
A dream widowed by modern medicine.
But there is no doubt,
nor will there ever be,
that to be a nurse
is to save the world
for their patience.

Purpose-filled dream
Save
The world.

SMALL IMPORTANT THINGS

Coffee, regular.
Two creams, one sugar, she says.
Smiling through stumbling speech
into her white hospital standard telephone.
Spiraled cord stretched
over the quilt her grandson brought in.
And maybe some grapes
or something.
Thank you dear.

Phone down she looks
right through me.
Now what were you saying doctor?
Something about a...
What was it?

I can't help but smile too,
and admire.

Where is this woman?
Not to be bothered
by some petty stroke,
the left arm she can't move,
or the whole of her left world
now missing.

God bless the small, but important things
like coffee
and grapes.

MIXED FEELINGS

A feared career's ending,
before it even started.

A career stalled on overambition,
now scented with the smoke of the dead.
The dead that now hang framed
at the very end
of a standard hospital hall
no one ever goes down.

Engraved:
*"Dr. Whatshisname
-Department Chair of who cares,
from a long time ago"*

Looking down on all
others who also daydream
of legacied name-sakes loosely tacked
on the backs of rare diseases,
only ever seen twice.

Seemingly enjoying every degree
of the lordotic necks looking up at him.
Sniffing their illusioned camaraderie.
Hearkening the good ol' days
of an era not yet gone.
A time of sweethearts, boy's clubs,
and doctors who smoked
and patted bottoms
because they could.

Or maybe he was different.
Now incompletely captured by a commissioned painting
Again,

no one
ever
looks
at.

Now sconced in peeling, rusting,
fading décor,
under flickering yellow light,
mostly out these days.

A broken wooden frame, worn
proudly like a washed-out letterman jacket.
Credentials stitched in silk,
like a real doctor.

RINSE. REPEAT.

Deep breath.

The kind that cracks your back,
all over.

Nights and days, and days,
blend together.
A continuum of sleep-deprived exitings.

The snooze button.
A savior,
but only once.
Found by muscle memory
with eyes shut,
but never fully closed.

Coffee.
Scrubs.
Self still anchored firmly
to the closest soft surface.
Bare feet
in tandem with eyelids,
reluctant to leave the carpet.

Shoes on,
Teeth brushed,
No turning back now.
The enormity
of the memory
of stress,
just starting to flicker
from the burning out bulb
no one's allowed to see.

Knowing you'll be here
doing this exact thing
only more exhausted,
tomorrow,
and the next tomorrow.

A rinse and repeat
without a rinse.
Equal parts
déjà vu' and déjà rêvé.

Dark to dark,
day to day,
week to week,
on end.

Then home,
to comfort the glinted bulb
and smoldered wick.
Feet reuniting
with their soft companion,
just minutes before
eyes close
and reopen seconds later
on their continuum
of sleep deprived exitings.

UNPREPARED

Nothing prepares you.
Nothing could.
For the tone,
its utter absence,
and the feeling
of those tiny fingers in yours.
The way they roll,
and fall
off yours.
Nothing prepares you for that.
Nothing could.

Nothing could prepare you
for seeing something so small
centered in a room
that engulfs it.
And nothing could prepare you
for the stillness of the air
that suddenly you can't breathe.
The air you wish
you could give away.
But that's not how this works.
And nothing
could have prepared you for that.

Nothing could have prepared you
for the look in her mom's eyes
as she watches yours
watch the EEG.
Their dark emptiness
as if life had left her
as well.
All things equally still.

It's times like these
that your soul goes missing,
time stops,
and things lose their meaning.
It's times like these
that nothing prepares you for.

Nothing could.

AND THERE SHE WAS

"Compress at a depth of 2 inches" they say.
Hospital gown down, chest exposed, leads attached.
Bare.
Surrounded by 10 people,
10 more in the hall,
and 10 more on their way.
Completely vulnerable.

This seems so unnatural.

Would she have wanted it this way?
Like a machine.
A chaotic, noisy, and messy machine.
More concerned with the process than the patient.
More with the heartbeat,
or lack thereof,
than the woman that surrounds it.
If she only knew how it would turn out,
how she would go.

"STOP COMPRESSIONS"
"PULSE CHECK"

… no pulse.

"CONTINUE COMPRESSIONS"

Feels like punishment, for her.

Crack.
An unnatural crack.
The kind you can taste.
With each forceful compression, a piston through her chest.
"Be warned" they say.

"You will crack ribs" they say.
But no one warns you about the sounds.
The moans.
The gasps.
The violence of resuscitation.

But your job is to compress, at a depth of 2 inches,
and feel, with no depth at all.

"STOP COMPRESSIONS"
"PULSE CHECK"

… no pulse

"CHARGING"

"CLEAR"

Her shoulders jolt forward, head back.

"CONTINUE COMPRESSIONS"

Shouldn't we cover her a little?
Why does she have to be so exposed during this?
I don't think she would have wanted to go this way.
…………
"Time of death 0200."

And there she was,
and there I was.
The inhuman admiring the human.
Both lifeless, and exposed.

SUNSET

Two fingers!
Can you show me two fingers?

Orange yellow sun, strong
through the blinds to my right,
warm on my face.
Surrounded by white coats
with blue masks,
saying things.
There, but not there.
Where am I?
Why is it so hard to breathe?
Beep

Can you give me a thumbs up?
Show me your thumb.

Sun's still out
but not as bright.
Short clips of choppy silent films
play out around me in flickered sepia tone.
Each ending with a beep,
then I wake up again.
A passive character
in an even shorter film.

Can you wiggle your toes for us?
Open your eyes.

I can see the sun is setting.

ODE TO THE INTERN

Dear Intern,

We see you.

Hands at ten and two,
belly fertile,
with face framed by crumbs of humble pie.
Busy toes just wet from
the system we swim in.
Still looking both ways before
crossing your T's.
Too in shock to hear your
soft loud inner voice repeating
the word "regret."

But should you find time
to look up from your trench,
you'd see us at your back,
because we've all been there.

Welcome.

PIECES

Lay there,
like you now do so well.
Perfectly.

Here we are.
This romanticized situation
of doctor and dead.
The after-fight
that moves slower,
with care and
lunch breaks.

Another *found in alley*
track marked to hell and back.
Now again lay supine at the
mercy of everything else,
while I, the hopeful pessimist,
confirm the picture on the
puzzle box,
and throw away the rest.
Walking away every evening in
consequential withdrawal.

Until tomorrow,

when I return
to picking up more pieces,
to throw them away.

SURPRISE

Hospital Day 2 of 17.

It's pronounced *gee-yan-buh-rey syndrome*,
I tell her.
A fancy French word for nerve disease.
She with her spiraled note pad,
scribbling notes for the family.
Me with my patient list,
folded, and then folded again.
Digging my heals in the batter's box,
preparing my saddle.
Readying myself for the dailiness
of his care.

Hospital Day 17 of 17

Last breaths always sneak up on you.
Talisman to the life it ends.
Homaged by silence.

TETHERED

Eyes roll and gesture
to the room
at the end of the hall.
The one with the soft walls,
no sink, and audible lighting.
From under its reinforced door
radiates a tethered cord of radical thought
rooted in reflex
and emotional incontinence,
stretched beyond recognition,
piercing the attention of few.
Frayed reasoning atrophied by hopelessness and pain
on a bedrock of neglect,
waiting for the next sterile human interaction.

THE WAY WILLOWS FALL

She sleeps,
vigilled by a daughter
inseparable from the life
now dissolving in her palms.

Fingers calloused by years
of motherhood. A trade
they both shared,
in a love story told
one meal at a time.

Bones filthy
with what-if regret.
And hope
bought with prayer
bought with fear.

Haunted by a quiet she's never met.

Each second
an unfair trade for the next,

while death takes its time.

Her eyes,
the way willows fall.

A CHILD OF DEAF PARENTS

No! He said. *Never.*
As a child of deaf parents.
Eyes, ears, closed tightly.

He refused to trust,
Scared but soon prepared, and he
Died in that red hat.

Breath short and labored
All alone on his island
Surrounded by boats.

THE LUXURY OF SHAME

Little do you know
or likely care,
but I'm scared.
Not for my life,
but because you know my name,
and you saw me last time.
And I could see your eyes roll
before the ambulance arrived.
After the pill bottle opened,
but before I woke up.

You think you know what control is,
but have no idea
until you lose it.

You see,
your days end in commas,
mine in periods.
You have goals,
I have needs.
Not a need to live,
but a need to die.

My only goal
is to curl up tightly
and die
in the dark ink at the center
of the period that ends my life sentence.

A full stop.
Quiet.
Calm.
Only then can I breathe deeply.

You
have the luxury of shame.
A life you take for granted,
with both length and depth.
And I
am doing my best
to plan my last breath.
To go quietly
at the end of my sentence.

NOSTALGIA

-nostos
Homecoming.
A familiar place
of comfort
and warmth.
A place of welcome.
A sacred place.

-algos
Pain.
Equally familiar.

The combination
fitting perfectly the dark mornings
still not fully awake
or present.
Drowsy mornings
spent feeling like you just fell asleep.
Like today is no more
than a continuation of yesterday.
Living on coffee,
graham crackers and peanut butter.

But now to rest
in the still of the quiet,
and the comfort and warmth
of a sacred soft bed.

And as it is
the moment eyelids touch
another piece of you dies
with the pierce
of the moment's worst possible sound.

Your pager
sucking the air
from the bottom of your lungs,
and keeping it from you.
Killing any calm you felt
for that brief second.
Depression folded on exhaustion
folded on defeat.

A painful homecoming
to a place
you never fully left.

CALL ME WHEN YOU GET THERE

Like clock-work.

Always asking
to be called "when I get there,"
and followed by
the obligatory nod and "will do, mom."

Never given a second thought.

And as I leave these beige walls,
overdressed with the stock and stereotyped paintings
lining the halls of this hospital,
a hospital I'm scared you may never get to leave,
after a hug I fear may have been
our last,
I recognize
the taken for granted
is no longer granted.

And that as I drive home
I wish
I had someone to call
when I get there.

COMPLICIT

No pitch, no hum.
No pomp.
No ceremony.
No clean cut sculpted
lines still warm from the patient before.
It's time to call it what it is.

Because by now
you should know
there's a ghost behind each of us.
Each recognizing the other
for what they are.

Aren't you tired
of complicitly chasing flashlights
into needless dead ends,
feigning concern for the journey,
and never dare speaking of
your unequal parts
psycho and somatic?

But you know it,
and I know it.
And so do those
that stand behind us.

FOR THE LIVING

There is no such thing
as pure stillness,
pure quiet,
deep breath,
until the first night
after being told
"There's nothing else we can do."
"I'm sorry."

But the slowing is gradual.
First breath, then sound,
then days.
And things lose their identity.

First things to me,
then things in themselves.

Hospital sheets
from itchy
to cotton
to nothing,
and my room
from confining
to holding
to dark.

What will be the last thing I see?
My wife?
My doctor?
These walls?

Will it be painful,
or will I die in my sleep?

In pure stillness
and pure quiet,
leaving these walls
for the living.

FOLDED

It's ok to start your morning
holding their hands,
telling them you care,
and that you
will do all you can to help.
It's this piece of human business
that should be done first.
Before picking up
your growing list,
folding it in half,
and starting the circus of your day.
Each medical record number a receipt.
An "I was here,
until I wasn't"
carved in ink.

The ICU can be a dark place.
Each room hued
by the memories of its prior tenants.
Each beep both a blessing and a curse
to all who hear it.
Beeps that sync
if you listen long enough.

And in the halls
there is forward energy
that fights a determined undertow.

So,
it's ok to start your morning
holding their hands,
telling them you care,
and you'll do all you can to help.
Because after taking your day's list
and folding it in half,
it's too late.
The undertow has begun.

APATHY OF CHRONIC DISEASE

Another vasculopathy.
Another drinker.
Another poor decision-maker,
with seemingly little regard
for the lengths people go to
around them.
Little gratitude
for the work it takes
to keep them alive,
from killing themselves,
despite their best efforts.

We all know their names,
their faces,
their stories.
and their decisions,
or at least we think we do.
From weekly visits
and leavings AMA.

The effort now
lies not in the care we give,
but in the care itself.
Its presence
and its intent.

CONFESSION

His spirit,
once bright behind
a church pulpit,
shone on Sundays, now
sings slow gospel to
regrets that sputter
and spit and feedback
behind the secrets of
closed eyes,
while worry hums melody
an old song,
rotten with silent confession.
His once tall, strong frame
now lay in complete mercy.
Each second baptized in time,
pausing for the chorus.

THE SPACE BETWEEN

Dim room.
Wife, son
daily updates.

Each exam shorter than the one before.

Goals of care.

He's a fighter, they say.
His heart is strong.
We're not giving up, they say.

They see a heart still beating,
I see eyes fixed, for days

What makes up this space?
The one between their hope and my acceptance,
between his heart beats and his fixed eyes.
Is this the space where fight lives
or a place for compassion?
Am I misreading the writing on the wall?
Am I the only one who sees it?
Or did I write it?

Am I the only one
not seeing
the fighting in the rooms all around me?
Am I the only one giving up?
Am I the only one not fighting?
Should I be?
After all,
I see no towels to throw
or white flags to raise.
And success stories exist for a reason.

Miracle is a word for a reason.
Right?

But his condition doesn't change
by the aptitude of my attitude,
or does it?

Or should I consider
that the person I am responsible to
and responsible for
is the same.
And this may not be the time
for towels or flags.
and that I might be the one
who occupies this space
between hope and acceptance,
and maybe I should join the fight.

RHYTHMED ONE

I don't expect
you
to get it.

Comfortably
standing there.
Smug as all hell.
Held up by the starch of
your oversized white coat
and equally mocking ego.
Poking dying people.
I can feel your
suede-lined pockets
from here.

Let your hands rest.
Your insulting injection of
big no-one-else-knows words are
lost… here…

You lost me when
you acted like this
was tough for you.
You.
Speaking dumb to the reality that
you're going home tonight,
concerns bubble-wrapped and
leather-stitched.

Please,
know.
The rest of my life
lies still by my side.
His snare no longer keeps

its rhythmed one.
The shine of his smile,
now a whisper song.
Growing restful
with impermanence,
readied for the backslide.
Hat doffed to time well spent,
and homesick for anywhere else.

INTRACTABLE

Here, again.
A well-known intractable,
on a first name basis.
And again,
here crashing her own party.
Her own show and tell.
Attention drunk
toasting to noncompliance.
A crime accessorizing itself.
A problem more software
than hardware
Each discharge portending her next return
as an incorrigible
reliable intractable.

STANDARD OF CARE

There's a place
where bodies parted by thin white sheets
tell stories
behind still lids,
where breathing machines hush
the now quiet crowd of what
once was,
where right and wrong are hidden in proper form
sterile procedure
and standard of care,
and where pupils grow more opal
by the day.

There is a place
where love stands still,
bedside,
in shared silence,
hand in hand with its better half

WHAT MATTERS MOST

How do you tell a wife of 63 years
a son of 60, and a daughter of 58,
that in times like this
what's most important is holding his hand?
It's ambient stories told
by familiar voices,
and him knowing without knowing
that he is loved,
adored and embraced.

ROOM 1

In the before,
John was a Navy man.
Now 51 years aged
since his blackest polished shoes
last kissed the sands of the west coast
and the salt of the pacific
dried under his eyes
for good.

6 years sung to sleep
by the brush of white waves
and creaking steel.
Those crested swells
still sing for him at night.
Softly.

His soul exists there,
in whole part,
starboard with a brotherhood
people don't understand.
Men who left their lives
when a number was called,
and the reason to live was changed,
and the reason to die was changed.

Reasons soon changed again
with the laughter of
his grandchildren,
who don't understand why he cries
while they walk around
in his blackest polished shoes.

John was a Navy man,
humbled by the myth

of welcome-home confetti.
His hands never left the glass,
its grip,
or its love for him.

Wife and child,
wife
and child.
Semi-formed shadows of
an unsavored past
traded for solitude
and the slurred memory of
nights with every star
in the company of those with
called numbers and
same reasons,
sharing their sea-brined summer skin.
A love shaded differently
and shadowed in uniform.

He no longer argues God's role
in those he killed
or those he loved.

Now coming to an end,
he readies his vessel for its last
night out.
An old two-seated, two-paddled rower,
more patched than anything else he owned.
Thin-fingered nails wrapped tight
around the neck
of the only trust he has left,
and the sweet bitter blur it gives.
Less and less,
until every star comes out,
and he is starboard again
with the numbered few
who know.

Sitting unsteadied,
waiting for the last drop
to signal his end.
A bow to the sea
and its darkest polished black.

ROOM 2

Mary is a writer,
whose life's debris waded
in scribbled plots and crinkled storylines
under a cloud of all-consuming
slow-moving, oozing,
loving companionate smoke.
The intimate haze that crawled
into every crack and crease
of her inners and outers,
filling every cell with embracing content.
Each tuft spooked and unfurled
into the next.

Cells falling fast
asleep in their own soft grey pillow,
connecting each to the next,
to those elsewhere,
and back to itself.
A one and all embrace
with every pull.

Sipping each down
to the last crumb,
the warm cool of every
breathless breath
paying homage to the one before.
Temporary on its own.
An end in itself, without edges,
until there was.

Deaf, blind, and dead
words landing on passive ears
but never staying long enough
to settle.

As whimsical as the smoke that kissed
her lungs for decades.

Years added and taken away
in weighted story
as futures passed,
thin hair and fickle veins appear,
fingers stain and ivory cracks.

Resolute to defend their origins.
To follow for now.
A blinding mark of denial

Nothing is better than the last one,
as she sucks her soul back in,
tapping the spent ash from the
tip of 50 years in subconscious preparation
for today.
The day the steroids stopped working.
The day the smoke won.

A day she will no doubt remember
hazily next week sitting benched
hospital front
enjoying her next last one.

ENTROPY

He ended it,

finally,

after months of subtle artifacts
and recoiled calloused words
broken on the mandibles of fellow
cliff-sitting note-pushers.
Empty threats and hollow points.

Old hopes now look
from his newly made temporal release.

Desperation now lay limp
with quiet eyes and
knuckles sprinkled sanguine,
powdered grey.
Coughing up calm blood and
bright red dignity,
while the healthy ration their breath.

ABSENT

I missed
what you told me
with your absence.

For years.

THESE TALKING HALLS

These halls.
These long, pale beige hospital halls.
Lined with human-shaped lifetimes
of untold stories
sung to sleep by the ever-present
rhythmed beeps some call life-support.
Cared for by the blurs of those
with someday plans.
Each signing out to the next fresh shadow.
Each an end in themselves.
of compassion fatigue,
then apathy

Like a wave
breaking the one that comes after it

And anyone who says there isn't
is either lying
or already too far out to see.

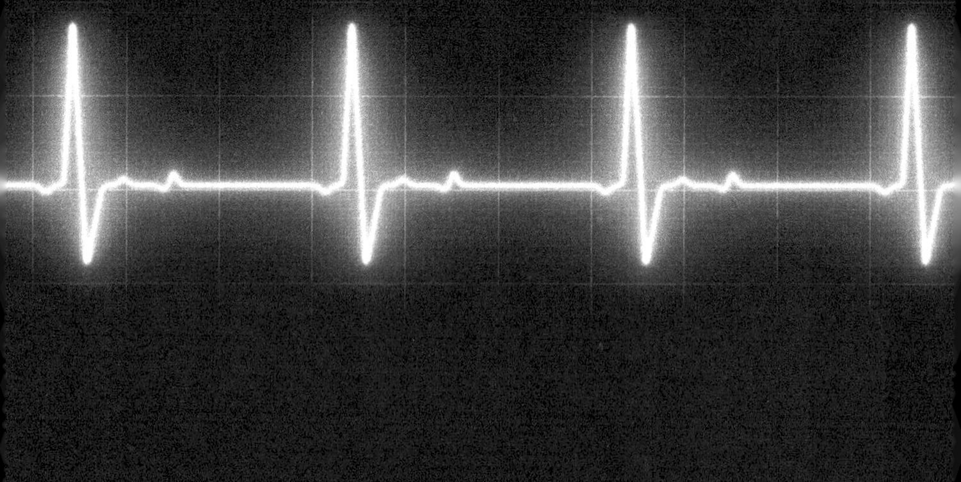

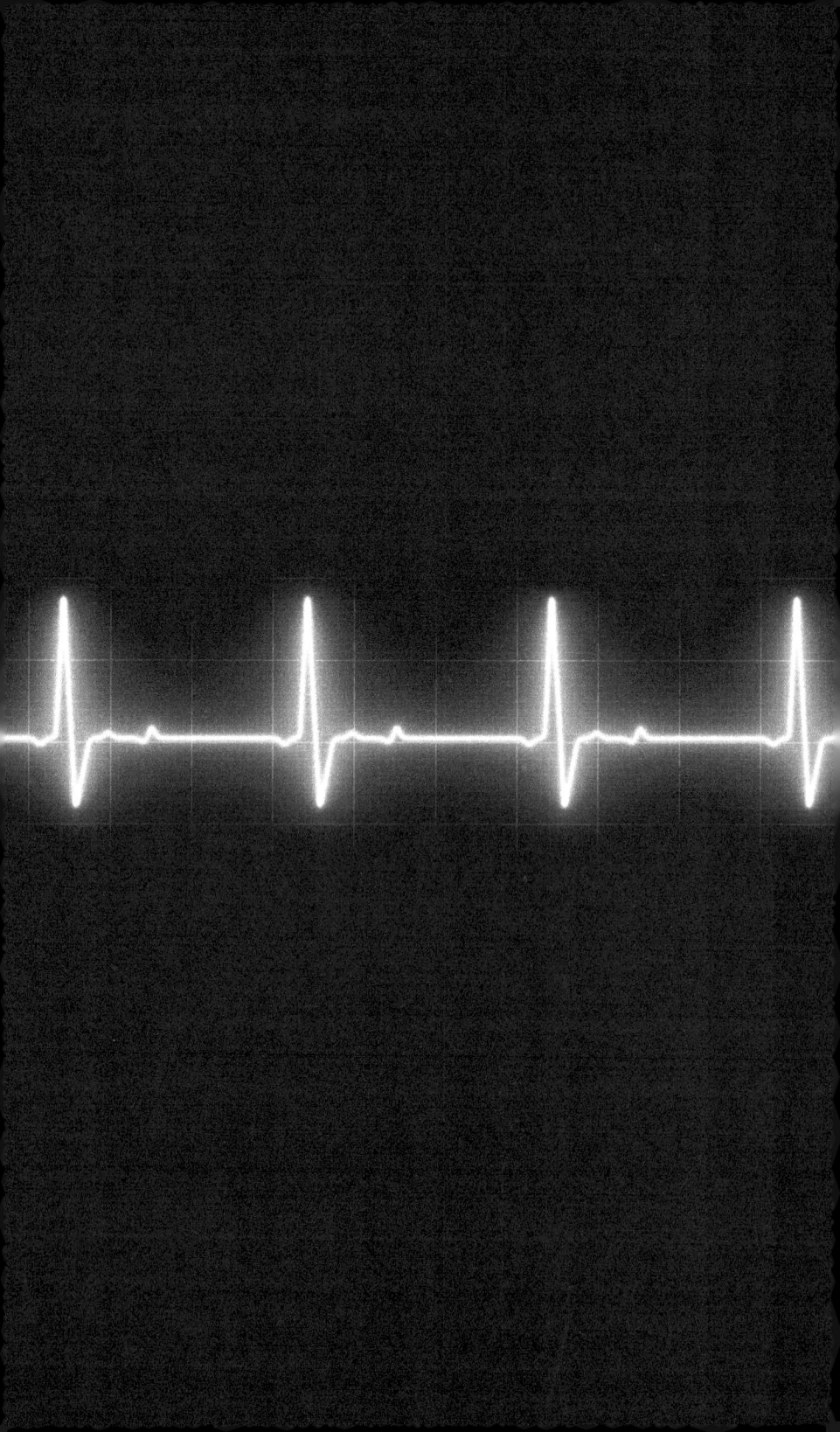

MICHAEL WYNN D.O., FAAN

Michael Wynn completed his neurology residency and vascular neurology fellowship at Oregon Health and Sciences University. His poems have appeared in *Akitsu Quarterly, The Cortland Review, Halkuniverse, Hektoen International, Intima, JAMA, Journal of General Internal Medicine, Neurology*. He was a poetry contributor at the 2019 Bread Loaf Writers' Conference. He is an invited speaker on Poetry and Neurology for the American Academy of Neurology's annual meeting and reviews poetry submissions to *Neurology*. His chapbook "Bodies of Evidence" (Finishing Line Press) was published in 2015.

His poetry explores the connection between the human condition and the natural world. He is fascinated by the randomness of nature and disease. Michael finds poetry to be uniquely suited to expressing the interplay between loss and beauty; between what is and what humans want.

Michael was a logger before entering medical school. When not seeing patients or writing he works on his log cabin.

ADVICE TO MY YOUNGER SELF WHILE MAKING EVENING ROUNDS

Es ist Vollbracht, "It is Finished"

Her son is empty as a shell on the beach.
When you explain why he won't survive
(helmets only do so much)
without the Lethe-filled braid of IVs,
remember, his mother is your patient.

Covering for a colleague, when signing out, do not say
"Mr. Jones is not my patient, but…"
On this Friday night Mr. Jones
needs you the way
fading embers need
a fleeting breeze to reignite.
He is your patient.

Keep up with the literature. Gather your ancestry.
Introns and exons are the rosy-fingered dawn
and Achilles heel of our DNA.
You must appreciate this.
Your patients will not.

Looking at a brain MRI—
its butterfly glioma
crossing the corpus callosum—
reflect on Julius Caesar's resolve
the moment before he crossed the Rubicon.
Your patient is waiting.

On your way home, as geese
warp and weft through indifferent clouds—
listen to Bach.
Someday you will be the patient.

BEING RECEPTIVE

Receptive aphasia is a language disorder where those affected have impaired or no understanding of what is said to them. Their own language production, however, is unmoored.

Good morning Mr. Smith.
Three chickens. My shoe, yes.
I'm here to help you with your language problems.
Pears.
I see.
The Sea. The wine-light sea.
I'll write.
Quality time in Purgatory.
A writer! A respected profession.
Ant's wit. Wait.
Antiquity.
Since.
You've been writing for a long time?
Molecules. The Man wants
some of us sick, others he wants
writing.
You sound like a poet.
Derek told me everything is a mess,
except language,
which is everything.
That makes sense Mr. Smith!
Then nothing. Empty wells
fill with night
but there's always more.
Good attitude Mr. Smith.
Lilacs.
Lilacs!
Oh!

EVENING AUTOPSY

Still as a fossil—
he's ticked off after 40 years
of booze and too-easy heroin.
Shocked red hair, pinched expression,
and eyes shut tight as rusted hinges
give him the look of a burned-out leprechaun
who lost his pot of gold to a smart little girl.

Dissolution is the resolution for his anger.
His molecules, aristocrats every one,
caring not a whit when his brain
said I'm done, will fall from him
like defeated ash from a distant volcano.

From some corner of this blue tiled room,
Elvis.

> *Are you lonesome tonight?*

What will all his carbon-based tissue
be in ten thousand short years?

> *Does your memory stray to a brighter sunny day?*

Under the weight of indifferent cities
he will be a tiny diamond.

IT STARTS WITH THE BRAIN

Half.
Hemi.
Two hemispheres scribed
by fold and furrow,
the primal font of the gothic novel
What Hath Evolution Wrought?

Two bound together for the One—
our gray planet from which everything
begins. All of it—

Hemingway's *The Snows of Kilimanjaro*,
violin partitas on Tuesday mornings,
AK-47's,
blue Mazdas, the Pantheon.

All of it relentless as the yellow
cotton dress falling away
on an August afternoon.

Insistent as Dante's comedy
extoling illicit love.
I am Paolo.
Next Thursday's barista—Francesca.

All of it.
In every circle and sphere.
All.

OBSERVATIONS OF A FIRST YEAR NEUROLOGY RESIDENT

New white roses
in the hospital gift shop
every morning.

Walking across campus
in the middle of the night
after seeing a delirious patient in the ER,
I saw Jupiter and Saturn
in the southern sky.
They were not that far apart.

Under our skin
we all carry the same
shades of red and loss.

Medicine is art.
The trauma nurse's clogs
remind me of Jackson Pollock's
Shimmering Substance.

When I'm on the pediatric neurology service,
at the end of the day
the sunsets
are all in a shambles.

Our molecules do not care about us.
Lest we forget, we behave
like we don't care about them.

The half-life of loss
is life-long.

FOUR PIECES OF ADVICE FOR NEW NEUROLOGISTS

1.

A demented patient remembers more
than she has forgotten. Remember this.
She will forget to remind you.
Focus on the picnic she had
with her love under the Chestnut tree—
iced tea, peanut butter pie, Verdi on the BBC,
then listen to her describe her scars
from her days in the Women's Army Corps.

2.

If a patient is older than 85 talk to him
like he is 105
or 30. Even better, listen.

3.

Mr. Smith is angry at his stiff leg
and right hand tremor. His language
is brutal as a medieval flag
carried into battle.
Imagine the gibbous moon
rising over Agincourt, the field
all black arrows and scarlet ego.
October mist rises and swirls
flowing with easy purpose
over the newly dead
without deference to lineage.
Mr. Smith wants to move like that.

4.

You are as full of promise
as a not-quite-ripe lime.
More than knowledge,
what you have to offer your first patient,
is ancient. A Bristlecone pine.
Be ageless.

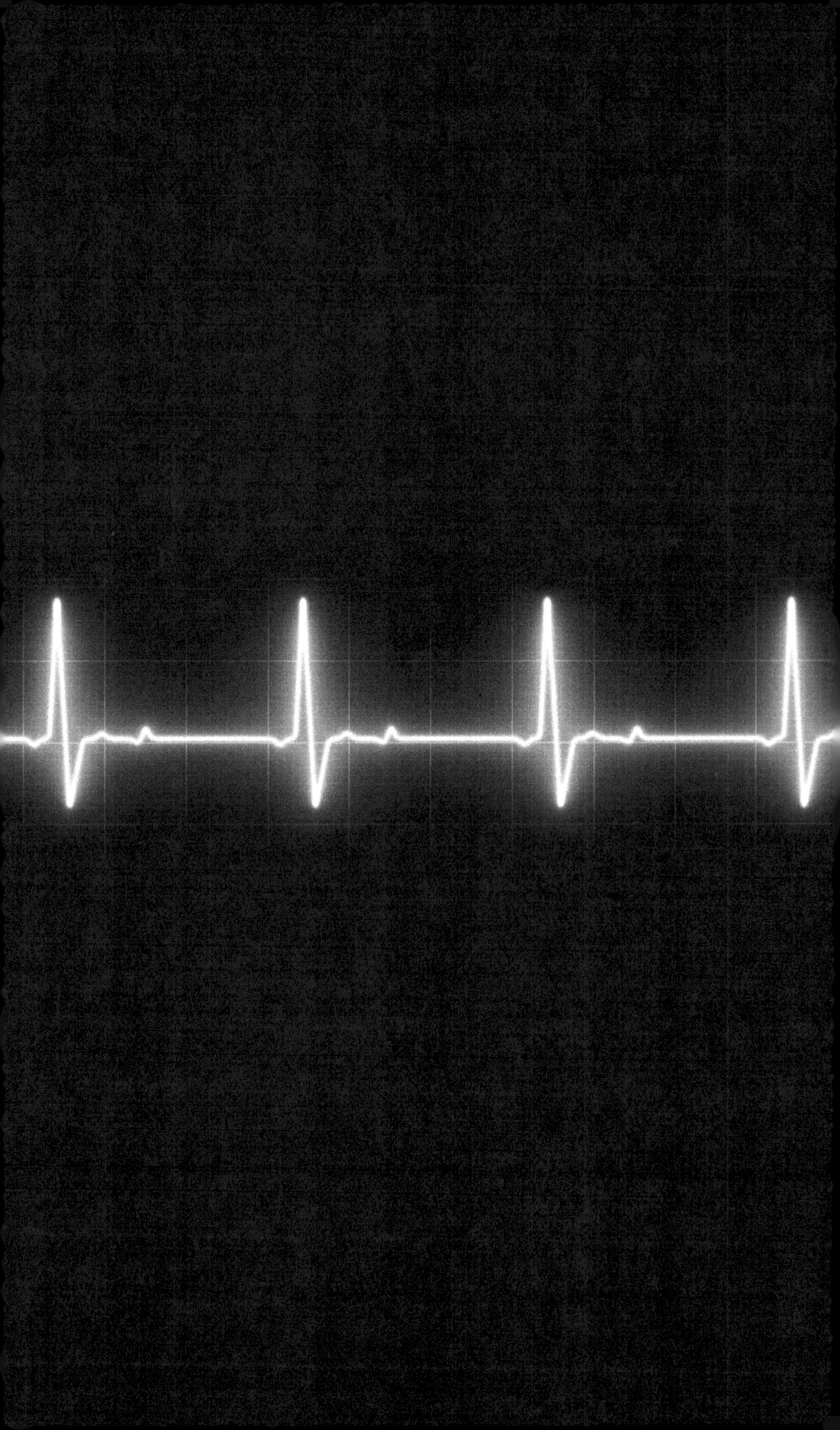

DOUGLAS HESTER M.D.

Doug Hester is an academic anesthesiologist in Nashville, TN. A reader and writer since a child, he pursued an MFA in Creative Writing after completing his medical studies. Learning about the medical humanities as he went, Dr. Hester has incorporated creative writing into his academic life via workshops and lectures for physicians and healthcare providers. Patients and clinical encounters influence his work, as writing can be a way to process difficult experiences in the hospital setting.

FIRST CASE WITH ADÉLE AND AEGIS

We lie awake in opposite corners
Of the house. Your babbling crescendo
Calls me to fetch your bottle. The dog
Waits until I'm in the nursery before
He comes yawning, settling near my cold toes.

I feel your body smile as we sit in
Edenic dark, our fingers wrapped on the bottle.
You stretch, knocking the unwanted formula
Away. The dog muzzles up the trickle
As your wet face pushes into my neck.

The hospital awaits, and I must leave
To put other people's children to sleep.
I set you down. You wiggle in the crib,
Fingers fumbling at the pacifier.
You sigh and roll on your side with eyes closed.

The dog knows to go, but I linger on,
Grateful you let me meet you here again.
The ORs might run past bedtime tonight.
If so, I promise to come tomorrow,
Another warm bottle in hand to give.

But it's what I'm taking that scares me.
The hall light makes my shadow tower over
You as I back away. I wonder if
Today I will do you harm, drag your heart
Out of Eden with my imperfect love.

SPRAYING COTTON IN BOLIVAR COUNTY, MISSISSIPPI, THE SUMMER FOLLOWING MY FIRST YEAR OF MEDICAL SCHOOL

The John Deere wheels cut hard coming to the turn row
that runs along the county line near the evergreen
copse in Paradise's south forty acres. In the wake
of the tire tread, a dull patch flashes within the white blur
beneath me. Exposed bone blooms among lobed leaves
of cotton. Five vertebrae lie bleached and unstrung.
I idle the machine, lurching to rest as diesel fumes
rise in a dirge to these remains at the field's edge.
I stand to see better. They are lumbar (without facets
for ribs) but unknown. All bones being the same
beneath skin. I have seen others, too: a woman's,
this past fall. The instructors started us on the spine.
Stay removed, impersonal. Yet intimacy surprised me,
cracking open her cranium, lifting her brain from its vault,
guiding my hacksaw down her forehead, between her eyes,
through her nose and lips and buckteeth, stopping when
the blade touched tongue. Dozens of muscles clung
to the skull, and it took weeks to tease them apart.
We only spent a day on her back. There are neither
education nor glory in vertebrae. But brains have blood
pulsing inside, cycling furiously in our imaginations.
Spines just stand and do the heavy work of lifting
without recognition, like this stranger. These bones
make a good monument. Brains would not last long
in Mississippi heat. Below my cap, sweat cuts down
my dirty forehead—glabella, the anatomists taught
me—and into my mouth. I taste the salt and dirt
of this old plantation, and know this field will remain
in me when I leave in September. I taste myself.
Evening looms, illuminating this shadowed past,
another crop of cotton, and the moist soil dissolved
in my blood. I shift the tractor in gear as cotton bolls
swallow these bones with a tongue of snow.

BREAK-IN

After the burglary—
when surgeons scraped
scalp from cranium, drilled
through skull, unearthed dura,
and raised tumor from
the temporal lobe
with stealth—you woke
from propofol and asked
me to hold a coffee
while you pawed through IV
tubing, your gown, blankets
soiled with blood and betadine.
Your hands snatched and grabbed
on the stretcher because
lost, here, somewhere,
lay the key to lock
strangers out of your
mind while you were gone.

AN INQUIRY CONCERNING THE NATURE OF THE CLINICAL EFFICACY OF PROPOFOL ON THE SOUL

Snaking through the transparent, saline-filled tubing,
the white mist swirls into your blood with
ephemeral whispers. Your cortex succumbs to chemical
promises of separation. I wonder: does your soul
hover as the surgeon niggles and tinkers, or does it
embrace the communion of solitude, carrying the flame
nearer your amygdala to burn in a primal country?
Here, the divorce is sudden, and we are left to think this
anatomy is you! We missed your light's furtive
release from this worn soul-holder, this crumbling
vessel of clay that houses your long-wicked candle.
Escaping through the cracks as the surgeon cuts,
you sojourn in shadow elsewhere, but will return
in time as the propofol ebbs from your blood.
Some emerge gleaming bright, anxious for reunion
after being away. Others pause at the abysm,
delaying re-consummation. How will you return tonight?
One candle here, I wait, burning myself. Ash and smoke
rise in the OR to greet the chary one who wafts back to
kiss the body: your soul folds in, like saline through a vein.

FINAL DIAGNOSIS

SO it's official, the freezer has a problem. It took six weeks, multiple appliance specialists and too much testing, but they did prove
                      my ice cream is not cold enough.

I thaw the taciturn repairman in six seconds.
What do you do, he asks.

                      I'm a physician, I say.

They gave me six months to live, but I know I was being killed by the medicines.
Thirty years later, I can tell you the secret of health is supplements
          and energy patterns
          and the secret is within us – the patients
          and doctors are dangerous.

I wonder what specialists touched him
          and what tests were done
          and how much time he spent without a diagnosis.
I work to reframe the discussion, hoping his discarded drill doesn't mar the granite.

I'm not religious anymore, but the power is within to heal
          and the deity is within all of us
          and gives us that power to heal
          and the deity has forgotten.
Our minds make us ill, that and food coloring.

So worldviews collide.
Models of medicine clash in the kitchen.

Health care reform isn't reform, it's refinancing.
Ending education at 5th grade
> *and legalizing marijuana and heroin will do more than this reform*
> *and euthanasia benefits us more than anatomy class.*

I liked anatomy, but tonight I learned the secret. The problem is in the freezer's mind
> and the freezer is an extension of the deity
> and the deity has forgotten
>> about my ice cream.

A MEDICAL PRACTICE

Thirty-six hours later, my pager rests,
done with another day and night and
day. Silence calls from my apartment's
kitchen. Inside my fridge waits this week's
casserole, a chicken mix of protein,
cream-soaked carbs and canned veggies.

I remove the last plastic spoon
from the box of white utensils labeled
"Elegant," peel back the aluminum
foil, and fill a bowl. I flick the top of
a cold Dr. Pepper can twice. The tab
lodges a dull protest under my fingernail.

I close my eyes. The microwave bleats
while I sit on the laminate counter
and bite into an apple. I eat over
a rusting, pleather card table suffering
in the corner. Borrowed instruments
lay before me on a wrinkled, blue surgical

towel: scalpels, needle drivers, silk ties,
and prolene. The half-eaten McIntosh is first.
I study the apple, pressing my ungloved
hand on the patient. The timbre and texture
dictate the route as thin tempered steel
cleaves tissue planes of apple skin

to tease the white flesh underneath.
The swelling below the surgical site widens
the gap. When cut well, the incision
glistens but keeps a dry field. I only damage
the underlayer twice. Satisfied with
apple work, I pull one pickled pig leg

from the jar kept for suture practice.
I slice the skin of the porcine model
to find tendons and bone staring up like grubs
surprised under rotting bark. I begin to tie:
running and interrupted; one-handed, then two;
instrument ties, left and right. No thinking

now. My fingers tug on fatigue and hold it
back. The skin pulls closer with each stitch.
I wet my fingers with yellow Palmolive soap
that mimics the blood from the chest of that
woman, the red-head who wrecked today,
her aorta sheared apart. Sitting here,

I almost feel her life washing over my hands
again as I throw knots. Soon, I turn toward
the only other furniture present: a mattress
waiting on the floor. I drop my pager
beside my dirty blue scrubs,
then reach for sleep to dull my hands.

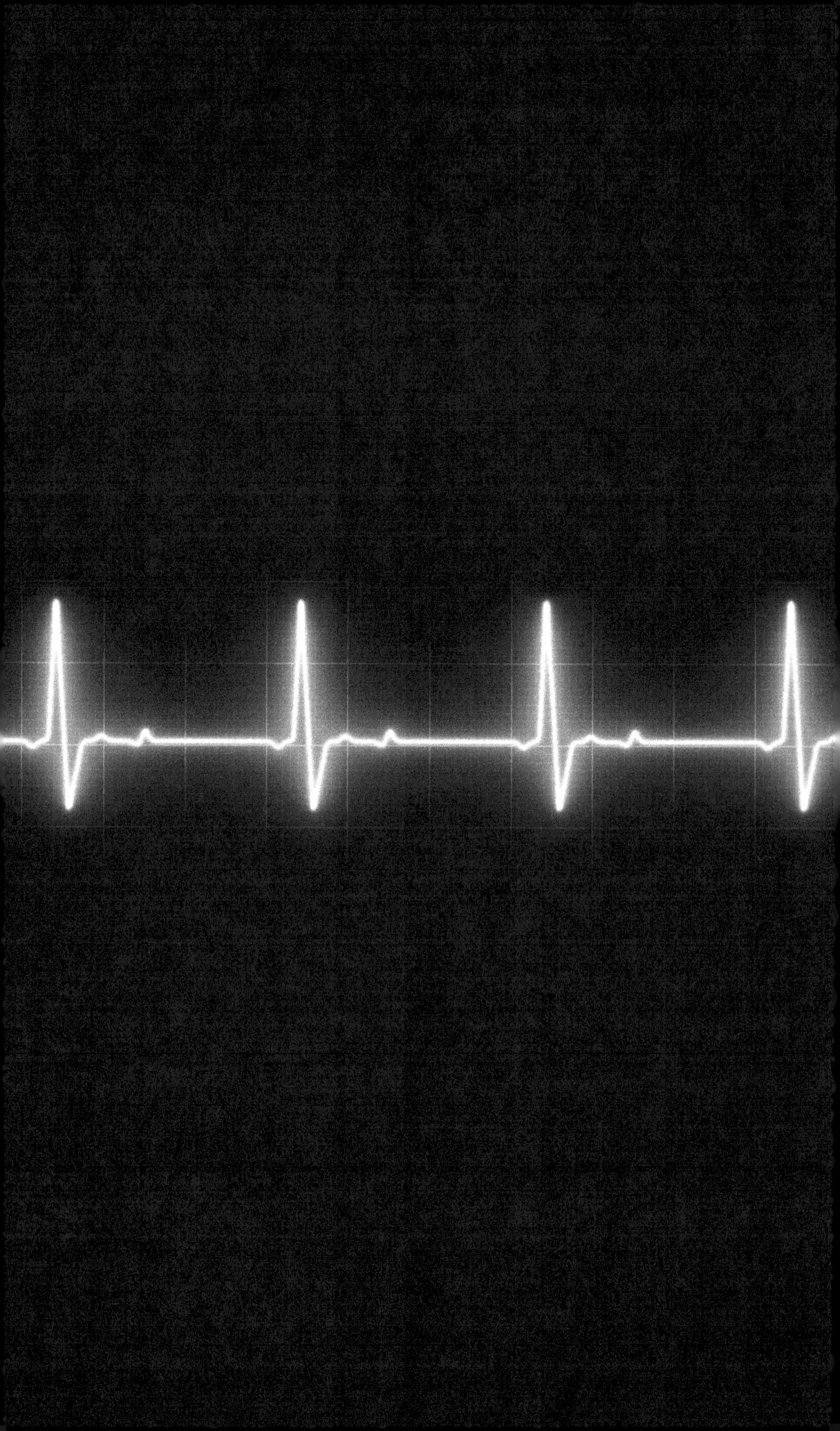

BRENDA BUTKA M.D.

During the five years between college and medical school Dr. Butka worked as a social worker, office worker, bookkeeper, waitress (including a stint in then-bustling Underground Atlanta), clothing sales, framing designer, and office cleaner. She also earned a master's in linguistics at the University of Michigan and finished pre-med requirements at Georgia Tech, which happened to be handy. Graduate training at Vanderbilt in internal medicine and pulmonary medicine followed med school at Emory, and she was on the pulmonary faculty at Vanderbilt for almost 40 years before retirement.

Her childhood writing career was spurred on by winning a world atlas in a Fruit of the Loom writing contest at age twelve, and a summer Hopwood award at the University of Michigan. Her poems have been widely published (*Florida Review*, *Threepenny Review*, *POEM*, *Slant*, *JAMA*, *Chest*, and others). She has self-published three books, and her paintings are also in collections around the country. When personal sloth and inanition threaten to take over, she thinks of an artist friend's motto: Either you do stuff, or you don't. And then gets up and does stuff. Mostly.

DO NOT RESUSCITATE

I can say
your father is dying.
I can say
wishing will not make it so,
belief doesn't change a thing.

I can say
love does not conquer all,
miracles are pretty stories told in church,
the movies you saw as a child are lies,
blind hope is not a recipe for success,
underdogs usually lose,
death is not the worst thing, it is just
the last thing.
But for you that is not true.

I can say
we have to pretend
that we can bring him wheezing
back to you like an old accordion,
chest pleating in and out,
singing his customary songs,
oxygen bumping its hurdy-gurdy way again
through his ancient heart.

But how can I tell you how
someone will shout down the hallway, kneel
frantic on the bed,
lean his fists against that old breastbone, sharp, frail,
one onethousand, two onethousand, and count it out.

I can say
we should not do this.
He will never be the same.
I can say
if it were my father.

I can say
do not confuse resuscitation
with resurrection, although
neither works particularly well.

You look like you are drowning,
pallid and slow in the waiting room's
underwater light.

So. Tell me.
Tell me again.
Tell me about your father.

SHIFT CHANGE IN BEDLAM

O little town, we turn towards home,
round-shouldered in our padded jackets
weighted with ordinary things,
totebags heavy with tupperware,
wallets and keys and cigarettes.

O little town, your moon
is not to be touched,
wrapped in a paper gown
of yellow fog. Your only star's
a cellphone tower, silent bedlam
blinking like a rat's eye on the hill,
the center of this doily of talk,
crocheted, frantic with longing,
from wavelengths we cannot hear
and do not understand.

O little town, so much is beyond us,
entirely out of reach. We call
and call the children, lounging mute, transfixed
in their pink and crowded bedrooms,
the electromagnetic spectrum held,
a careless gift, in their pretty hands.

O little town,
this elevator's full at seven.
Ward clerks and janitors wait,
cold and patient, until,
settled on the shuttle bus,
they reach out to lasso a familiar voice
from the spidery air, a small
bright thread to guide them home,
cellphones alive and warm.

O little town, your hallways and garages
bend in greasy light, clang like
a cage of hammers. Singing to herself
as she puts her purse away, this nurse
has spent the day tending
one or another fragile packet
that has slouched its translucent way
toward this bedlam to be born
damaged, too soon,
each turned in its cozy skillet
when the timer rings. Behind her song
in the parking lot,
darkness buttons shut.

TRAVELING LIGHT

"Pure energy, the nature of light, underlies all.
We emerge from and dissolve back into this radiant
ground. Not only can you know this-- you are this."

—Susan Morrow, translation of the pyramid texts

you are light, glowing like a candle
pale, waxy, ethereal, detached
and anemic, passive in the hospital wheelchair
heading home from surgery
back stitched together
with transparent thread
you are traveling light
carrying nothing, wearing
your one t-shirt, the stretchy pants,
the hospital's yellow socks

immersed, I suppose, since you
are not talking, in the shadow magic
of half-sleep (perhaps it is
a bright world you are revisiting,
or just absence,
eyes closed against the light)

I am trudging behind in my dark coat
the plastic bag with your shoes, your wallet,
your watch, your toothbrush, your instructions for showering,
not to bend, not to lift, to call
with a fever, your new aluminum walker
a urinal, pills layered in their amber cylinders

it's heavy work here, to remind ourselves
we are both traveling light, light traveling
a lit fugue made of recycled stars' breath
circling, combined and recombining,
glowing as we wedge you
into the front seat, support you
up the steps, heavy onto a kitchen chair
comets trailing light only as we come apart
in this dense atmosphere
parallel, traveling light unravelling

DEAR ABBY:

      I

Woman wants new, better life

She wants to say it's a virus,
a fungus, it will go away.
This time I'll save my money, divorce
the jerk sooner, be more
sensible, stay put, throw out
more anchors, fewer balloons.

She wants to say I was young
and pretty and chemotherapy
saved my life for many years.
I know I've been lucky, but not
lucky enough, there isn't another life
and I'm floating away.

She wants to say I want
a new, better life, but really
just any old life will do.
Tell me, how long do I have,
how do I look, I'll take more
vitamin C, what should we do?

      II

Woman wants new, better life

just not any
of the four
ex-husbands

not any
man in particular

not the couch
not the tv
not her lonely
house

is a rag
of sunshine
thrown on the floor
enough?

can she stitch
that rag
into a shirt
wear it defiant
every day?

III

Woman wants new, better life

run more
run less
smile more
don't bother
never smile
again

take this pill
unfold an epoch
of receptors, transmitters
dopamine everywhere
luminescent

eat kale
relax: eat chocolate
eat a flower, a nasturtium
find a baby to sing to
take lessons
feed him redbud

tell the family
to go to hell
save your money
get on a bus
sit next to someone
who smells

dream of reading
a longform poem
at a street fair
the crowd paralyzed
in wonder

throw away all those
old bills, tax forms
stockings, polyester
turn them into art
throw the art
away

stop talking
to the open fridge
unless the mayonnaise
answers back, then
transcribe

DIAGNOSIS: M. AVIUM, HEPATITIS C, CARCINOMA, THROMBOCYTOPENIA, HEMOPTYSIS

ribs, collarbones, femurs a nest of sticks
around his belly, a giant egg
held carefully in his skinny arms
taut as a drum
blood in the pink plastic basin at his side

he doesn't want to die
we can't persuade him that he will
he can't believe that we cannot stop this
thinks that if only we wanted to
we could do something
our white coats are no protection
don't shield us from his stubborn despair
he despises us for our weakness
our lack of will, our refusal
the shabby way we treat him,
a sick man
we stand on the side of truth, but that is no defense
here in this room every morning
he says Jesus is his only friend, and he too
was a carpenter
he says he might as well just get the bus
back to his mother's house
we have to agree
he can't accept what we cannot do
can't accept what we can, which is
to be there, to be satisfied with his contempt
which has to go somewhere, carrying his fear along
to touch his hand
to touch those fading bones
to get him home

CHARTING IN THE CLINIC

I spend all day translating bodies into words and back again,
stenciling pictures as abstract as the moon
onto your chest, into some form you might understand,
channeling you in braille, in one of eight hundred languages lost
in California, in the incantations of serology,
a kabbala of numbers, a web of dancing dots supposed to be your
heart. All of these things I turn into something else,
struggle to twist into a ladder, an alchemist's recipe, a rope for
rescue weave into comfort or at least a plan
to cope for a while with whatever might be
lingering outside waving its own semaphores which
I must admit, I missed entirely, so we both
are on our own.

You speak my language, you say, delighted
with the good news, affirmation of your exceptional self, when I
talk about bodily hyperawareness, a bit of anxiety which dates to
your bike wreck
or your pneumonia four years ago. I'm a seer, a shaman
to intuit that you're a little on the obsessive side, and, reassured,
smiling, no more appointments necessary, you head out
to the gym, satisfied , these fictions—yours and mine—
useful, and close enough to some truth to work for both of us.
I can enjoy my prophetic status for a moment, until I meet
the patient and her family in Room 12.
I spend all day, clinic time, sitting in a small concrete room,
a sequence of such rooms,
a plastic chair for you, whichever you is here
for this fragment of appointed time,
a plastic chair, on wheels, for me,
a tin desk, a computer wedged in the corner,
a keyboard, and here we sit, you
against the wall, my data source, my historian. I am here to edit

the story of your life, annotate the text
mixed of truth and myth transliterated
into your chart, your data dump, you as seen
from our point of view, refracted, redacted
thin-sliced by our microtomes of statistics and time.

What are you telling me, your gold chains and perfect hair,
your pedicure and good shoes? You go to Florida for the winter to
play golf. Yes, you have some friends there, but your cough
is always worse in your condo beside the clubhouse.
We're turning your story as best we can
into something that comes out with a moral,
a diagnosis, a plan, a place to go, an explanation,
a statement about the future. You want a crystal ball.
Your cologne is exclusive, you move inside it. Where
is your husband this morning? In that chair
across the room, looking like he wishes he were
holding your hand? Are you rescued? Or walled in?

I spend all day imagining how a bat would navigate
this hallway. I'm missing the gear, the ears, the sonar
but still committed to the flight. A dog's view would be quite
different, redolent with a deep history of where you've been, the character
of your own dog, someone else's pajamas, and might
tell us more than your own DNA sleeping in its tiny tubes
reeling off its encyclopedia of letters when aroused,
in a chant with its own interpretations.
Sometimes your only language is Cambodian, and your grandson
has no idea what the tattooed lines circling your thigh
in a blue sleeve really mean. He shrugs, says it is an incantation,
a lost script, an old language, protection. He says no one can read
it, even you. I suppose you have been
off to war more than once, but we cannot talk about this, your
grandson doesn't care or cannot know. But at night you do not

sleep, wake up gasping, want a pill, ask for something, believe in
magic.
I cannot imagine what you imagine as you watch me,
as you turn towards me in your plastic chair. I'm
putting everything I can into your record here, charting your voice
your heartbeat, your puffy ankles, the evolving fiction
which, for our purposes, will be you. You have created yourself
many times, rewritten your history, the meaning of those painful
prayers,
your truths ephemeral, volatile, but at least yours. Mine? Well,
we settle on a pill, shake hands, smile ineptly, acknowledging
our temporary and mutual good will, which I know is not enough
for nighttime with its knots of blood and its dark spells.
I spend all day translating bodies into words and back again,
sitting in a small concrete room, imagining how a bat would
navigate this hallway, interrogating your DNA, trying to sing along
with your current self, in a pentatonic scale only a dog can hear.

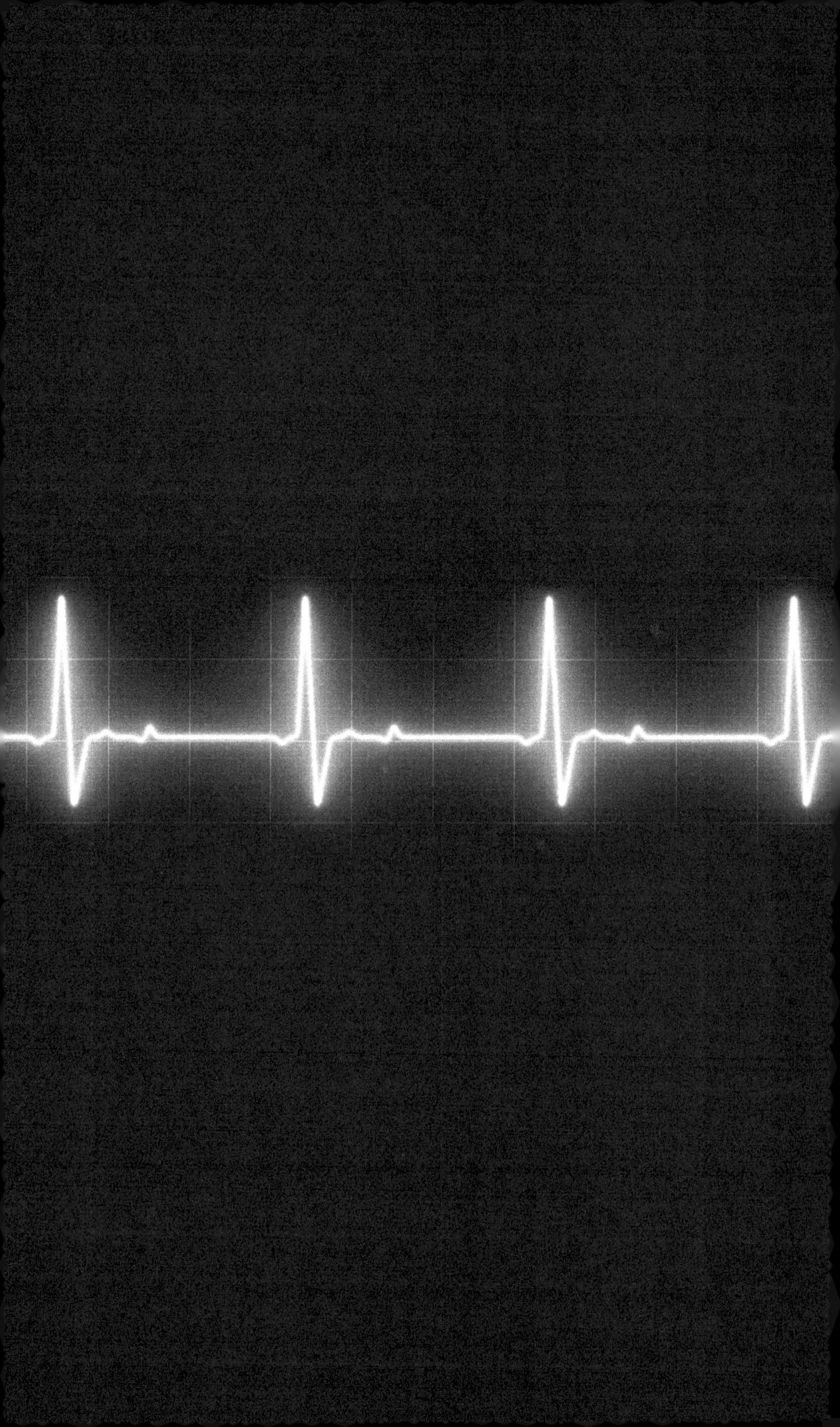

WILLIAM ROGERS D.O.

William Rogers is a pathology resident at Brandon Hospital, located in the greater metropolitan area of Tampa Bay, Florida. His path, unlike that of many other physician poets, started with poetry and later grew into physicianship. Born in Chattanooga, Tennessee, he completed a bachelor's and master's degree in English, before moving to Denver, Colorado where he taught Poetry, Mythology, and Composition for many years at the college level. As a teacher, Dr. Rogers continually encouraged his students to engage with life's seemingly unanswerable questions, as undertaken by the myth makers and storytellers of the past. He strove to help his students find their voice in the process of refining their technique. In this time, Dr. Rogers began moonlighting in the university cadaver lab as a teaching assistant—a job he loved and one that would ultimately shape his life's journey.

Though his passage to and through medical school was non-traditional, he completed medical school at Lincoln Memorial University and is currently training and brandishing a microscope to see cancer with his eyes in Gulf Coast, Florida. He is the author of a full-length screenplay, multiple short stories, and numerous poems, in addition to current work on multiple scientific papers. Like his journey to medicine, Dr. Rogers' poetry is in no way typical. His work considers and reflects on the harsh thoughts of the inner self-critic—truly, the things we don't say aloud. He does not shy away from the tough relationships we try to forget and the cringy feelings we try to avoid. Just as he always told his students: "Be truthful; the reader will know in a heartbeat if you are not." His poetry addresses dark themes, often with a rollicking wit that brings air to difficult topics, in an effort to let life be seen clearly, in all its full complexity, for what it is.

AGONAL

Watching you
thrash for air throwing
your whole body into breathing.
Yank out all your lines
pull off your oxygen mask
bleed all over the place and then
shit the bed.

Watching you
do it again and again.
Moan and throw the remote
at the respiratory therapist
as you gasp for the easy-breezy air
that is all up in the rest of them.

See, my lungs are trash too
and what am I gonna do
about any of this?
Watching you
it makes me want to go with you
wherever you're headed.

ELEVATOR POEM #9

i've never been one for the rat race. at dusk
as i was leaving the hospital, i handheld the elevator
for another in scrubs to feign kindness

one of the elevators to one of the parking garages, not
one of the elevators to one of the floors of the hospital

she thanks me; she smiles; she talks a lot; she says she can't
remember where she parked the car. Says it must be the third
or the fourth story. *boopboop* I hear myself say

press the imaginary car-fob button with my left hand
press the real elevator button with the other

she smiles, gets it, talks a lot more before the elevator bings
we hit the third floor. "Good Night," she says, smiling. then realizing
i only made the boopboop noise over our entire banter, i say

"Everyday is the Same Day." she snort-laughs, although this
isn't the occasion for a snort-laugh—or maybe it is—this brief
Godspeed shared

between strangers, between two people. she leaves to find her
freedom while I still gots many many stories to go.

IT'S OKAY, YOU'RE OKAY

You were the first. And now you're with me till the end.
Medical school ended last May. It's February now.

A brand-ish new year and you just coded out.
Already referring to her in the past tense.

Dead now for maybe two minutes, i fought tooth and
fucking nail for you and you died anyways. Regardless,

You're . . . sorry. Her . . . parents are down the hall waiting for the worst
news i might muster—with an aunt, maybe a boyfriend or a
brother—i don't know.

She's my age. She's 46. i knew her and i liked her. Just a couple
of months ago. Right before Christmas. You were here

for the same thing—tricuspid valve of her heart slathered
in bacteria, cocktailed by sharing drugs and sharing needles.

You let me be kind to you and i really needed that then.
She helped me shake the phony imposter syndrome for a bit

so that although i don't know what i'm doing yet, i still felt worthy.
i felt validated. i know how to offer genuine empathy for a bit.

This moment will overshadow the million modules and training
meetings on professional development i will ever do.

And so here, now, her Pastor Bob gawks in her doorway from the hallway.
Rubbernecker. She should have had more in life.

i remember watching a tv show when i was a youth—this tall
handsome, pissed-off white doctor says, "I only work with

patients that want to live today!" or something jackass and similar. This was before medical school, rotations, before residency, before

fellowship—any of it. And like this tv doctor's patient, she had been in
and out of hospitals for months. A few minutes ago, Karl was on me

hard. Busting my ass about going lower, pushing harder. i broke three ribs at least already—felt them go—and i kept going for more anyway.

And now you are the stillest thing in the room. Only a handful of months earlier
so alive and funny. Easy to answer all my questions. Politely compliant

with my physical exam. She was definitely Hospital Sick, bugs in her heart.
Word on the ward then, she was The Queen of AMA. Frequently flew here.

Now, a few months later, i didn't even recognize her, for the smut incessantly sailing in her veins—her physicality warped and faded

so abruptly. i had to see her chart. i literally had to
see my own prior notes on the computer screen from Christmas time

before i would know to believe it true. That this is you. And now you're gone
as our lives move on. Our time pressed. Our asses covered. Meanwhile,

some wild-eyed preacher lurks the hallway on tenterhooks behind the glass wall
to pray with her naked corpse. We cover her with coarse blankets

as he enters. Her doleful loved one's wait in the ICU waiting area.
We will sit with them. Tell them. They will cry.   The tv

doctor waits for the right person on whom to perform his smashing
indignant miracle, despite your undeniable will to not live.

i'll give it to you—you outdid a tremendous amount of education, training,
time, money, and the massive efforts of a collective of some sharp

and positively stubborn minds. Minds now stunned in our dumb nonplussed
state. She didn't want to be saved, one could say. Most of us are

more afraid of death than we are of living beat up, shitty, squandered
spiraling lives of poverty, monotony, isolation, and addiction.

When you and i were talking around the holidays everyday
i told you this would kill you. But you already knew that.

Should i have been harder on you is not the question . . .
And i am not in the mood to debate free will's existence right now.

i am simply asking the questions: What do you want a life to do?
Do you demand to save it or else? Was this finally supposed to be

The Event to scare her straight? This young weathered, brow-battered, pin-cushion,
now here, what, as something to practice clinical skills on like a dummy.

When is it enough to rid yourself of another? When is it okay to give up?
Why did I still push on you and push on and push on you? Karl screamed

at me amidst chest compressions: It's over now. She's done. Calling it. Stop.
Just Stop. Can You Not just friggin' STOP already, man? As it writhed spitless

lost last squirms, shuddering, shriveling, jutted, just as you go. What to make
of the shell of it lying exposed, on a hospital bed with godless lines and tubes

The madness of the machines irking it on with these most inhuman sounds.
When the ICU affected come—look not for a real or recognizable form.

Seek the haggard molt and pray for a soul that might or might not exist? her vapid marble eyes gaze up at the far far beyond—

it's okay, you're okay. i want to comb your hair. it's okay, you're okay.

Tell a person—relax, be at peace. Tell them it's okay—see what happens.
Try telling someone to stop fighting. Somebody who's already gone.

i am stiffled sick with the questions. And right now, if anyone, you're the only one,
the only one amongst us all, who really knows the answers.

SOME BIUTIFUL SWALLOW

—for Dr. Hannah C. Anchordoquy—

So, evidently; my great-grandfather fell
in the street in Cleveland, and he died
as his heart was sky blue and bad.

   My sister tells me not to tell our mother she told me any of this

Tale of the bastard who ran out on his tender wife
and child. So the slow suffering world
formally induces stenotic introductions

   Some shitty way to go, i say—Cleveland and all.

Now, He's all introducing himself in my life at 44
says He's coming for me.

   You better go, sis says, get checked out.

Nah nah, you're just some old, heartless man who ditched my
great-granny to Boompaah to Tennessee. Some long gone
flightless dead brute who makes new families all over the 1940s.

   Seriously though, I'll go with—what are you doing tomorrow?
   Meh, i say i'm ready to fly, sister, but really

i share no time with the sky lately i groan and moan on Politik
drone on—debt due to MultiNationalBank—drone on—my job—
due to be there by two—drone on— due to denigrating commute
drone on—due to Petty Congenital Lonely Defect, First Problems
entailing my ever-Worldly sad genitals, my achy-back Failures,

        and an ugly QRS complex.

   i tell my sister do not tell mom i told you any of this,

     but on my EKG

        there's a swallow

           i've never met before

PICK UP THE PHONE

The floor shines like the sun.
The halogens above, i guess those are
halogens. The moon is between our earth
and the sun tonight. New moon. No moon.
Black room. Should I call yet?

Mr. Giammalvo has been known to enjoy
our corridor as of late. Glassy-eyed stumbleena
ass out, wandering around like a goddamn
idiot. These are not pejoratives. Big moons
make ever bigger tides. Waves that can only trash.

The only sustenance at this hour in this entire leviathan of a
building vending machines; the only water flat like faucet urine.
Christ, what am i doing with the only life i know i get?
i am getting Mr. G. out of a pickle. Sir, please
let me help you. Do you realize you're actually in another patient's
room right now

Please, lemme help you, sir, please.

Never having worked third shift before and new
to this hospital, new to this career—new to it all right now—i'm like
        i skip lunch to go upstairs, stand on the helipad for a bit.
        i skip lunch to go downstairs, stand on the pavement for a
bit. Anything to study the moon.

He's not an idiot; his daughter was in from Denver just
a few days ago. Mr. G just needs a few sensory cues
aural or light or touch. i am getting paid to rip him
from the binding spell of delirium under fake corridor
lights, and who's to say i'm not actually the jag-off here

What if i'm delirious too—then who's in control?
It is easy to clean shit off the floor so it shines
again, yet, what mess is this. The moon, said
to be 4.5 billion years old. The doctor in charge
is angry that he has to. Has to do what, unclear.

Has to come up here to this awkward, blindingly clean hall.
To order other people who make minimum wage
to put restraints on Mr. Giammalvo. To travel
to the moon, knowing via car it will be a 130 day
trip. To ask another to strap down a fellow

traveler who is doing nothing wrong, except
for being lost on a different rock where they dance
stupit and the lighting's bad. Mr. G is screaming
now, and will scream all night, till the screams
clean to moans and then the moans slight to whispers.

Now distant wheezes and he's mumbling crazy shit
His daughter told me he's an astrophysicist—or used to be. Told me
to call her if things got Badbad. And right now, he gives off no light
Only reflects our own. Is it time? Please. Tear this heart out.
i hate the shine and pick up the phone.

HOSPITAL GIFT SHOP

we will not tell the children
about the impending surgery

instead we will buy ice
pops and paw patrol dolls

extend the denial—even outright lie
if it comes down to it. In nights, hold

the house within a quiet web of whispers.
we get Spider to babysit when she's not

at Publix, and when she works they'll sit
with me in the lobby where they got lollipops

and candy bar machines. Hospital Gift Shop
toys that spin and bark and shake for fun.

While at home, the dogs dodder heavy, sick from overfed
As the very foundation quivers. What season is this—

where doom bangs the shutters and won't stop
till we're all lost and you're done, my love.

CAN'T YOU JUST CARE

Care for them
Nonstop
To your own detriment.
Under duress
We applauded you and gave you
those two weeks of long

Mandatory ceremonies, where even our CEO came
So get back to work and hold any regular bodily functions for the rest of your career.
Cause you're lazy and immoral if you don't.

Can't you just care for them
Nonstop
To your own detriment?

No pizza for you till you break. No breaks for you till vacation.
No beach evermore. Close your eyes and tap your heels if you want to see the sun.
Go care elsewhere and don't stop, otherwise, go home.

And, your kids aren't our patients
Unless you're a hassle, ill-equipt, bad mom
You'll cut the kids in half. Find a way.

Close your eyes and tap your heels evermore. Find a way to do both: Run your home, manage your stuff, and be on time, which is late already. Brooms are for roadtrips, daytrips when offered.

So you used to shoot a solid three pointer; well, aces.
So you used to ice-skate like a banshee; well, wicked.

Nobody cares anymore.
We mock your grace.

Admin condemns your sighs.
Just do your job and care for them
Care for them all nonstop to your own detriment.
Care till you can't feel anything at all anymore.

RESCUE KIT FOR JUNKIE

Overdose Education not being synonymous with overdose Risk Reduction, the Naloxone given, the Naloxone done. upon leaving The Class, i went for the plunge

Three days later i came to in a sewer with mighty hulking voices jeering and crashing, closing in Then a mimetic flash, my two leechpets sudden in lights shown septic from wet trash,

Emesis, Ectoparasites and Defecation to boot, i can never say i remember flushing down a manhole. Then Hero-guy said, I found him (me). He is (i was) over there (here).

Here, Junkie is Over Here

How infatuated must a person be to force themselves down a slit in the earth, down the scariest, rancid abysm of a manhole to force unrequited rescue upon the

miserable. i wrote Here, Junkie is Over Here, Heroguy a letter and put it into a prestamped envelope. i can now gain closure, apply the relationship-building values garnered from my suicide

attempt toward re-socialization principles taught to me by my sewer mentor Harudo medicinalis if ever given the opportunity. But, i'm asking you now, why try for one who is ready to die

in the infestational sludge darkening all me and them Ectovermin. Harrow our light, come back out of a manhole. People need to do they stupit shit, so then our actions may cleanse

while these words do nothing but drop us further and further down into the distant clasp

RIDE HOME WITH ME LATER

For all of this
there is a reason
you say.

i'm not so sure anymore. Above
the warblers murmurate in flocks of jet-black

fire—sputtering and flickering—beat on a pale endless slate of
sick dead sky.

So, the cancer travelled, doc said, from his testicles to his
brain—from the Bottom to the Top.
There is no reason for such.

Who knew this could even happen?

i'm sorry . . . all the horrific things he said to you
especially near the end.
That was just the Big C talking
the pressure of the masses thrashing his brain.

Remember that one birthday when he got you the *Learn French on Audiodisque*
series—he sounded so stupit saying: *comme, je, son, que, il, état, être,* and *avoir*

He always did promise you the world.

To leave you under a flat unforgiving steely-mirror rude sky
Scathing lunatic birds
Now your windshield is all turds.

It actually feels like a funeral is happening today, dudn't it?

Ride home with me later, sis.
i'll wash your car tomorrow.

i know you know i never liked him.
you know i tried to.

i'm sorry . . . all the abhorrent things he said to you
even years before he got sick.
Decades before the transmigration of
the sickness from his testicles to his brains.

But, no really, i believe you now—no really, i do, sis.
Everything has a reason.

Murmuration has a reason
Even if zoologists—well, ornithologists, can only speculate to
theory—we know now

When loved one's gather
scrape together warmth, safety, and connection
despite all this tragedy

sullen and druthers,

it is truly a spectacular site.

PATIENT LOST TO FOLLOW UP***

Diagnosed on a Monday
Surgery on a Thursday
That's today

I don't think I can do this

God is love to you, doctor
But God hates me
I don't want you to take my member

When I was a child, I knew
Under the universe was a group
Of workers who kept cogs moving wheels which

Turns the sky from sun to night
And I saw donkeys and trains and later
Penises in the puffy clouds by day

In evening it all glistens
Busy miracle workers turn and turn
Me, dumb with wonder on my back in the grass

It was all quiet, except crickets and shit.
Now to survive my cancer
Requires these workers

It also requires my castration today.

Radical penectomy. It sounds like a punk band or a legal contract
Written by candlelight behind a door. Nailed now
On my back behind another door with a sign

That says *No Entry Without Badge*.
The workers and the donkeys and the trains
And the doctors in the holding area

Holding all us people about to be cut open
Or cut off. God's weird ways. Spare the
Staff. I Take No Comfort in Thine Rod. I can't

let them do this to me. I have a son who's six
And a wife—I finally found love. My life,
it's just beginning. Consider them.

Consider your family the tall doctor says.

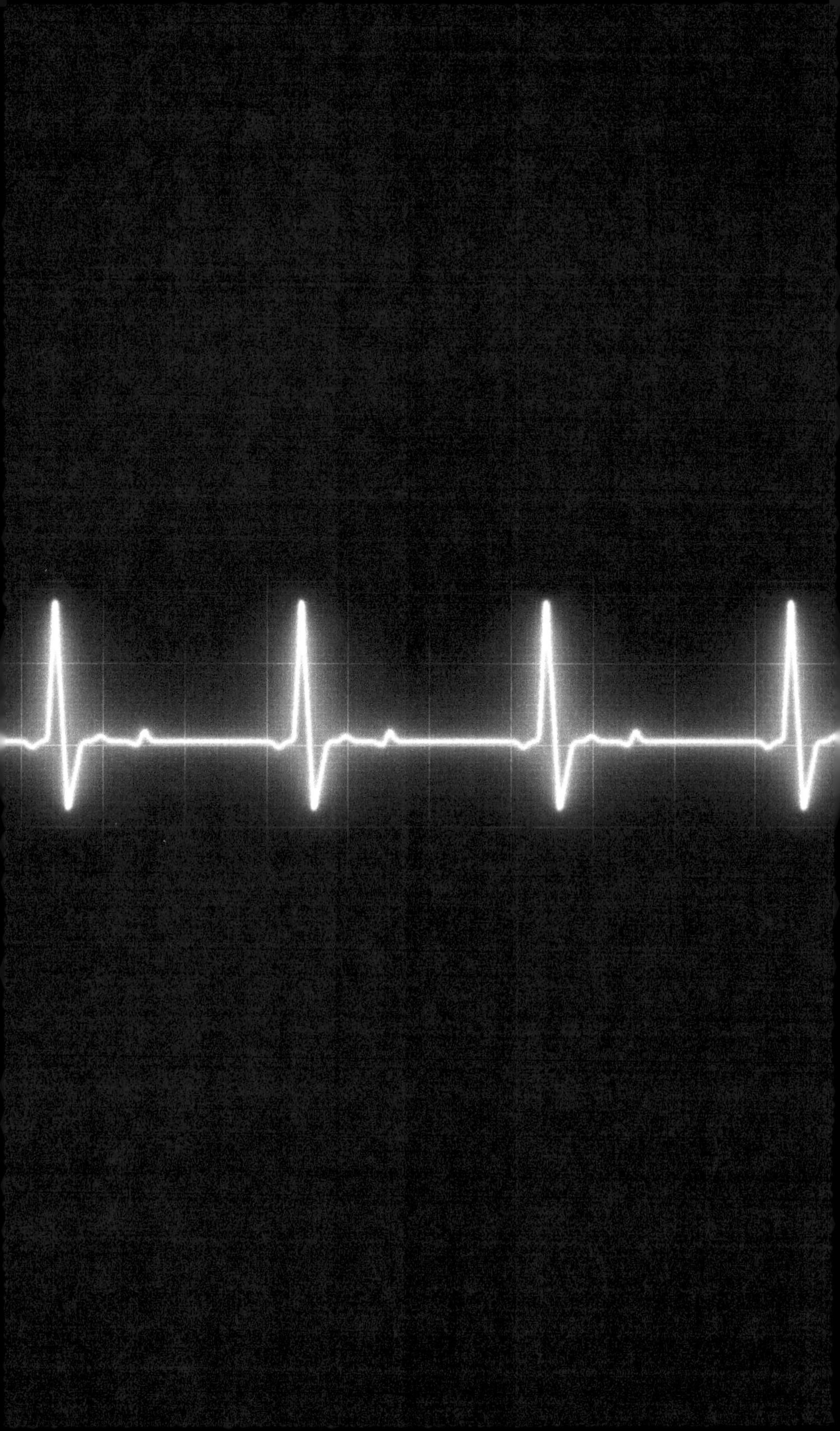

BRIAN CHRISTMAN M.D.

Dr. Christman is Professor/Vice-Chair for Clinical Affairs and Associate Program Director/Medicine Residency for the Vanderbilt University Department of Medicine. He also serves as Chief of Medicine for VA Tennessee Valley Health Care System with clinical focus in Pulmonary/Critical Care Medicine and Hospital Medicine. Most of his youth was spent in Tulsa, Oklahoma before four years in New Orleans for college. He came to Vanderbilt for Medicine residency and fellowship, eventually joining faculty. His poems are often based in the medical experience and underscore the contention that those of us privileged to be in healthcare should occasionally pause to reflect on the amazing people we meet and events we experience. He has published poems in *Annals of Internal Medicine, The Pharos, Chest, Vanderbilt Tabula Rasa*. When he is not caring for patients or writing he is often found inexpertly making furniture and turning bowls or visiting his young grandson.

CCU JAZZ

The windows darken
But she is lighter.
A weak lash blink, fingers grasp for traction.
Standard 4/4 breathing no longer suits her
A jaunty Joplin syncopation commences.

Her heart, always the diva, moves center stage
A Gilbert and Sullivan tach accelerates
Discordant PVCs, pure Bartok, demand attention
Abruptly she goes full Coltrane improv.

The house staff, strict traditionalists,
Will not allow experimentation.
After shock and awe
Amio hooks the intruder from the stage.
Blessed synchronicity returns
The rhythm becomes an ambient Eno.
Sleep is possible.

RESILIENCE

We guide through crisis.
Captains who know rivers
As their own names
And reach port, despite the storms.
But not today.

The old, new widow
Collected his few possessions
  -a smooth handled wheelchair
  -shave kit nestled on a plaid shirt
  -wrinkled photo, In dress blues
Before the long drive home.
Our even keel was lost,
Waves surged over gunwales
Tears down cheeks.

Time is short, others call.
We can waver, but not stagger
Like suspects walking the stripe
Before the bright torch of suspicious cops
Avoiding detection until balance returns
And the water is calm.

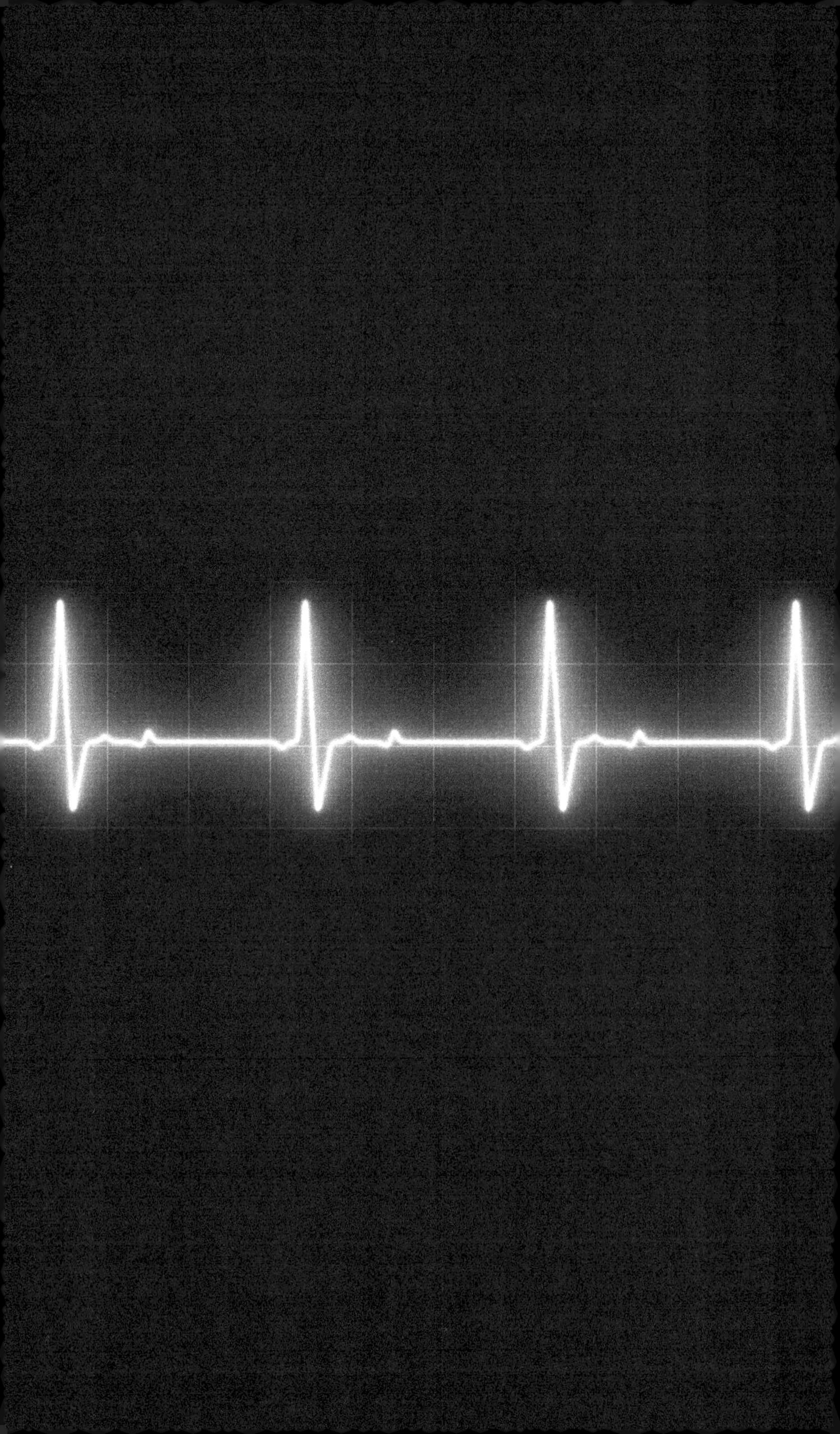

LEALANI ACOSTA M.D.

Lealani Mae Y. Acosta, MD, is an associate professor of neurology and a board-certified neurologist specializing in neurodegenerative memory disorders at Vanderbilt University Medical Center. After graduate studies in psychology and physiology at Oxford University, she completed medical school and neurology residency at the University of Virginia. She completed behavioral neurology fellowship with Dr. Kenneth Heilman at the University of Florida. She also earned her master's in public health at Vanderbilt University.

Her clinical practice includes caring for those with memory disorders. Most of her research revolves around cognitive impairment and Alzheimer's disease, including clinical trials for new drug therapies. She is also a clinician educator, which includes serving as a College Mentor for the Vanderbilt University School of Medicine and as behavioral neurology fellowship director at Vanderbilt. Her range of publications reflects varied neurological interests, including peer-reviewed research articles in cognitive and behavioral neurology and creative writing. Her publications have appeared in *Neurology*, *Neurology: Clinical Practice*, *JAMA*, and *JAMA Neurology*. She also has published visual arts, including fiber arts replicas of prominent neurological historical figures, such as the brain of Albert Einstein and a model of Phineas Gage's skull and the tamping rod.

SPAGHETTI WITH RICE

My *lolo* (grandfather) ate spaghetti with rice. A fork stabbed the slippery tangle of noodles bathed in Prego, oily pools of red-orange sauce seeping into the mound of pearly white grains, spooned in concert.

Rice was everywhere in his, my parents' homeland. *Too hot, too far, too crowded,* I bemoaned.
Fried rice with Spam, swimming in a golden yolk of sunny side up egg for breakfast, rolled *lumpia* (eggrolls) filling threatening to burst the rice flour wrappers, even flippin' dessert was made of rice

In the kitchen, the squat box, bigger than I was, held levers of a magical rice slot machine.
I would pull one down and a cascade of rice
    tinkling down the chute to the drawer below --
        the sound of raindrops
            hitting a broad banana leaf plucked for shelter
                on the way to school
or so my parents said. *Why didn't you just use an umbrella?* I wondered aloud.

My patient gazed at me earnestly, sincerely. "I'm so glad you are my doctor and were able to come to this country before coronavirus would have prevented you."

Can he feel the grass strands of the walis-tambo *broom sweep my parents' kitchen?*
Can he hear the rasp of coconut shells scrubbing the floor?
Can he smell the waft of jasmine steam billowing from the rice cooker?

I yield a reflexive, stiff smile, partial pearls. The smile reserved for when everybody else around the dining room table roared with laughter while I waited for my sister to translate the joke as relatives would cluck, *Bakit hindi siya nagsasalita ng tagalog?* (Why doesn't she speak Tagalog?) My parents tell me I refused as a child, stubbornly insisting, *I'm an American.*

Thank you, I hope my English is good, because it's the only language I know
What did you say? ...I'm sorry, I don't speak [insert Asian language]
No, I'm really from Washington, D.C.
My parents are from the Philippines.

I squirm in my starched white coat while, in my mind's eye, I see my grandfather eating his spaghetti with rice.

The hospital gown
uniformly shrouding
all well ill still clothes

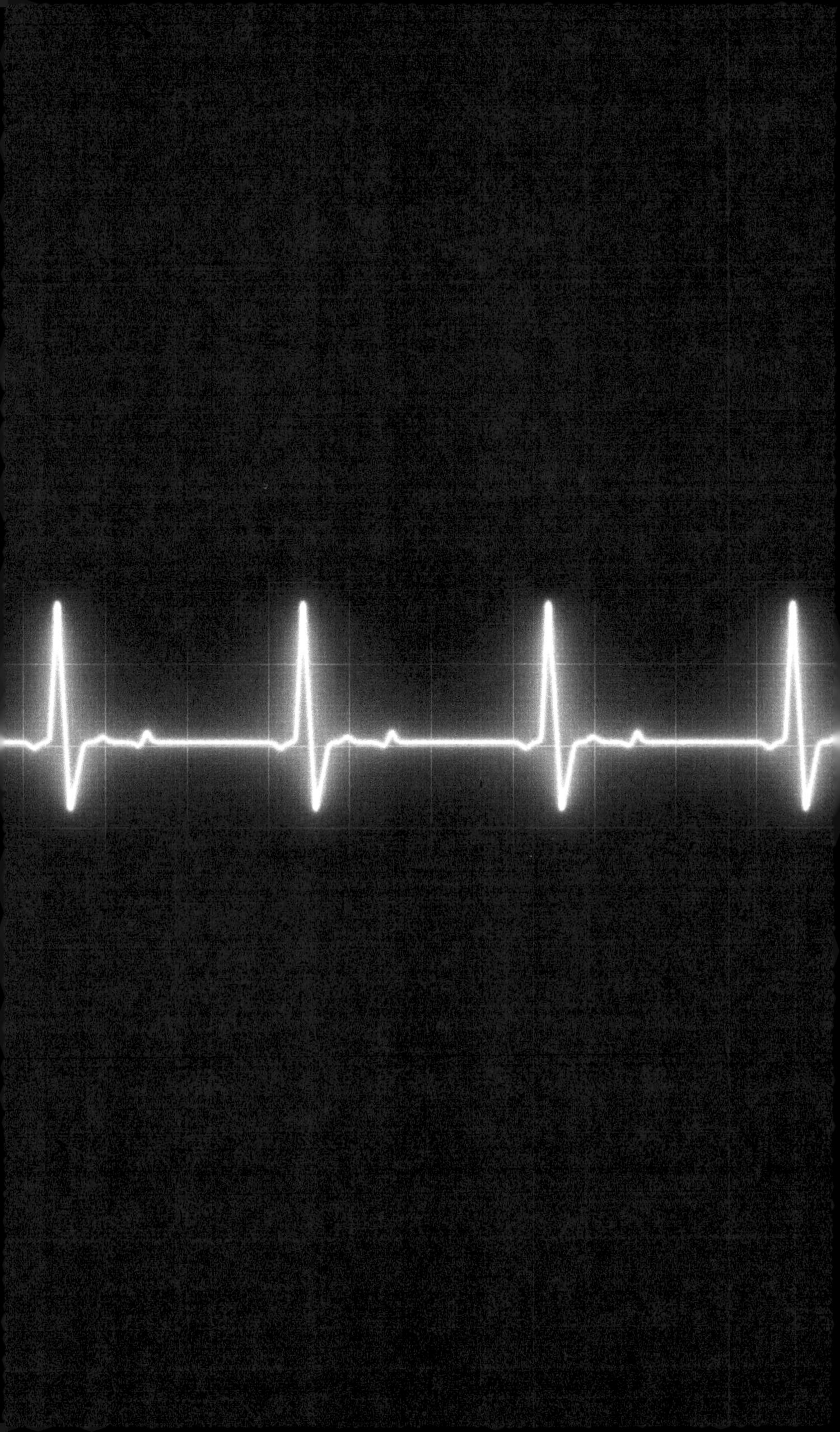

VEENA KUMAR M.D.

Dr. Kumar is a neurologist, singer, writer, and mental health advocate. She grew up learning Carnatic (Indian classical) music and playing violin. She first developed an interest in medicine in college at Columbia University, where she majored in ethnomusicology and biology. She completed medical school at Emory University followed by neurology and epilepsy training at Case Western Reserve/ University Hospitals Cleveland. She now practices epilepsy and general neurology in Pennsylvania.

Dr. Kumar suffers from bipolar depression, diagnosed in medical school, and it has colored her medical career thus far and drawn her towards poetry as a means of healing. Her writing has appeared in Doximity Op-Med, The Styloid Process: Literary Journal of the Emory University School of Medicine, and the Columbia Science Review.

While on a medical leave from residency, she self-published a book of poetry structured around the different facets of the disorder via musical metaphors. She hopes to continue to capture the emotional landscape of medicine through writing.

THE SCENT OF COLLAPSE

I just want someone to tell me
"It will be ok"
that I don't have to feel the pain
of my patients anymore,
that I don't have to collapse
under the weight of all that suffering
just because it's my job.

IT'S CHRISTMAS EVE

It's Christmas Eve
(there are these songs that are in my mind)
Told a man his cancer is back
and it's Christmas eve
I told him and I didn't even sit down
(and now I can't get these songs out of my head)

I cried to my dad when I realized what I had done
who am I and what
am I doing in this world
The things I do impact other people
and I'm not ready for that
These are real people
they have families and loved ones
I ruined this man's day today
and it's Christmas eve.

LIFE

In the hospital bed, cold and unresponsive, he is extubated.
I stand in the corner, head bent in reverence.

Family in a circle, praying.	Psalm 13.
Smooth jazz, playing.	His favorite music.
Daughter, saying:	"Our quiet hero."
Wife, hands shaking.	His face in her arms.

The beeping stops. Quietly, he slips away.
At peace.

RESIDENCY

An endless *chug, chug,*
not a race but
a slow grind.
I wake up and wonder
how I ended up here.

Sometimes it seems *important*
what I do;
later gets lost in mundanity
in doing what people tell me to do
lost
in feeling like I don't know.

Clinical practice
is always so *different*
from textbooks.
I have stopped worrying
about asking stupid questions.
But there are some things
I can't ask.
Every time I mess up,
I think:
what is the point
of the hundreds of patients
whose reflexes I have checked
when I still can't get it right?
These things take a lot of skill,
practice,
but why does it take me
so much longer?
I have been doing this now
for 6 months.
6!
I don't know anything!
At least I know that I don't know?

It might not seem like a big deal
people are dying, afterall,
but how can I keep doing this
when I feel so incompetent?
How can I save lives
with an imposter syndrome this heavy
even despite
the things I have achieved?

MR. X.

Mr. X quietly walked into the Transitions of Care clinic, checked in, and took a seat in the waiting room. As he looked around the room filled with patients, he felt a sense of calm: he would be taken care of here.

This was not always the case. During his last hospital admission - something about an infected knee - he had been bombarded with young eager faces looking at him and his knee like he was some sort of circus animal. For this reason, he had a general mistrust of the doctors especially those in the short white coats. But he had been to this clinic a few times and there were only long white coats and smiling faces and people who seemed to genuinely want to help him. Last time they had even procured a cane for him, seemingly out of thin air.

Mr. X was homeless. For the past year, he had been living at the cemetery, because he had found that no one bothered him there. He lived off of bags of Lays potato chips. Every time he ended up in the hospital, which was a lot, he was told he was malnourished. Although he had been homeless now for two years, he felt a sense of shame every time he had to admit this to a new person. It branded him as a lower class of human being. There were many factors contributing to his homelessness - a lack of education, unemployment, but mostly it was his heroin use that had emptied his wallet and sent him to the streets. He looked forward to telling the doctors he had been clean for a month. Even so, the itch to use again persisted.

Here, they did not judge him, and for that he was grateful. There was a nice case management worker who had tried to help him get into a shelter last time and helped with paperwork for Medicaid. He hoped the case worker was working today.

Mr. X suddenly realized that he was holding a clipboard and looked down at the sheet in front of him. Anxiety swept over him; he was a slow reader. He often told people his vision was bad to avoid the embarrassment of telling the truth that he had only gotten to 8th grade. Slowly he filled out the form, hoping that he was doing it right.

He was starting to nod off and tried to focus on the television to stay awake. He had walked an hour from the cemetery to Grady and he was exhausted. He had only ridden the MARTA bus once, and it had been such a confusing experience and he had ended up in the middle of nowhere. He figured he must have been standing on the wrong side of the street, but how was he supposed to know? He wondered how normal folk were able to figure it out. Maybe they used their phones. Mr. X didn't have a phone. He knew that riding MARTA would make his trip faster and less painful, but he just wanted someone to come with him and show him how to do it.

His elbow was starting to hurt more, too - he hoped one of the doctors here could help him. What were the names of the medications he was taking? He had forgotten. They had run out long ago. He should have written it down. As he contemplated this, feeling especially stupid, he heard his name being called out by a pretty lady in blue scrubs.

It was time.

CITATIONS

DR. DOLBOW

Dolbow JD. You Know I Love You, Right? *Neurology* (Humanities in Neurology) 2021;96:287.

DR. HESTER

Hester D. Break-in. *Neurology*. 2018;90:745.

Hester D. An Inquiry Concerning the Nature of the Clinical Efficacy of Propofol on the Soul. *Anesthesiology* 2014; 121:661

Hester DL. First case with Adèle and Aegis. *Anesthesiology*. 2012;117(3):669.

Hester D. Spraying Cotton in Bolivar County, Mississippi, the Summer Following My First Year of Medical School *JAMA*. 2021; 325(3):310.

Hester D. Final Diagnosis. *Anesthesiology* 2012; 116:222–3

DR. BUTKA

Butka B. Do Not Resuscitate. *JAMA*. 2012;308(16):1613.

DR. WYNN

Wynn M. Respectable. *J GEN INTERN MED*. 2022 (37):1300

Wynn M. Advice to My Younger Self While Making Evening Rounds. *Neurology*. 2015; 84 (6) 629

Wynn M. Being Receptive. *JAMA*. 2022;328(17):1773

Wynn M. It Starts with the Brain. *JAMA*. 2021; 325(23):2406

Wynn M. Observations of a First Year Neurology Resident. *Intima* Fall 2022

Wynn M. Four pieces of advice for new neurologists. *Neurology*. 2020, 95 (15) 698